TYPE
B

Eat Right 4
Your Type

PERSONALIZED COOKBOOK

Eat Right 4 Your Type

PERSONALIZED COOKBOOK

**150+ Healthy Recipes
for Your Blood Type Diet®**

Dr. Peter J. D'Adamo
with Kristin O'Connor

Photographs by Kristin O'Connor

Previously published as *Personalized Living
Using the Blood Type Diet® (Type B)*

BERKLEY BOOKS, NEW YORK

THE BERKLEY PUBLISHING GROUP
Published by the Penguin Group LLC
Penguin Group (USA)
375 Hudson Street, New York, New York 10014, USA

USA I Canada I UK I Ireland I Australia I New Zealand I India I South Africa I China

Penguin Books Ltd., Registered Offices: 80 Strand, London WC2R 0RL, England
For more information about the Penguin Group, visit penguin.com.

PUBLISHING HISTORY
Previously published in eBook format as *Personalized Living Using the Blood Type Diet®*
(Type B) by Drum Hill Publishing LLC in 2012
Berkley trade paperback edition: October 2013

Library of Congress Cataloging-in-Publication Data

D'Adamo, Peter J.
  Eat right 4 your type personalized cookbook type B: 150+ healthy recipes for your blood type
diet / Dr. Peter J. D'Adamo with Kristin O'Connor; photographs by Kristin O'Connor.
    p. cm.
  ISBN 978-0-425-26947-3 (pbk.)
  1. Diet therapy. 2. Nutrition. 3. Blood groups. 4. Naturopathy. I. O'Connor, Kristin. II. Title. III.
Title: Eat right for your type personalized cookbook type B.
  RM219.D29 2013
  641.5'631—dc23
                          2013021043

PRINTED IN THE UNITED STATES OF AMERICA

10 9 8 7 6 5 4 3 2 1

Cover design by Jason Gill
Cover photo by Christopher Bierlein
Book design by Pauline Neuwirth

Contents

Type B

Soups and Sides

Type B

ix

Introduction

Let food be thy medicine,

and medicine be thy food.

—HIPPOCRATES

FOOD HAS THE potential to heal and strengthen our physical bodies, support our recovery from injury and illness, and potentially change our genetic destinies.

Not only does food provide sustenance and nourishment, it provides an opportunity for creative expression and community, whether through developing new recipes or ways to prepare a certain food or in sharing a meal with others. When I wrote *Eat Right 4 Your Type* in 1996, I explored the connections between blood type and diet, and outlined specific nutritional programs for each blood type. Since its publication more than fifteen years ago, I have continued to research and write about the role that foods play in our lives, and I have tried to create support materials and guidance for people who follow the Blood Type Diet.

In 1998, I wrote *Cook Right 4 Your Type*, which acted as a handbook for my readers, providing recipes, cooking tips, and planning guidelines to help navigate the process of food planning and preparation. I always wanted to take this further as I felt there was an aesthetic quality about food and food preparation that should be reflected in a book, not just with great recipes but also with beautiful, four-color photography that celebrates food. About three years ago, I met Kristin O'Connor. Although she came to see me as a patient, our conversation turned to following the Blood Type Diet, cooking, food preparation, and the work she was doing as a personal chef, food stylist, and food blogger.

I was impressed by her dedication to nutrition and healthy eating and by her ability to simplify the food-preparation process, which for some people can be quite daunting. Over the ensuing months, as we worked together as doctor and patient, our conversations returned again and again to food. I felt that I had found in Kristin the perfect person to collaborate on a book project that would blend the scientific concepts of the Blood Type Diet with the artistry of cooking to create visually stunning cookbooks specifically designed for each blood type. Kristin has a passion for the Blood Type Diet that is unparalleled, and an encyclopedic knowledge of the food lists for each of the blood types. She is creative and resourceful, and she appreciates and respects the need for food to both taste delicious and be nourishing.

For the past year, I have been enjoying the recipes included in the books, and I have to say that I've been knocked out by how delicious they are. They are also easy to prepare, as I know most of us have limited hours in the day for food planning and preparation. The recipes contained in these books are suitable for individuals or families, as well as for special events and entertaining. Additionally, there are helpful food preparation tips, suggestions for how to organize your kitchen, food storage guidelines, and suggested resources that can make meal planning and preparation easier. My goal has always been to provide accessible information that is easy to incorporate into daily life, and I believe that Kristin has accomplished this.

These cookbooks represent new food and healthy lifestyle possibilities for my readers; they combine the science behind the Blood Type Diet with Kristin's expertise not only as a chef but as a believer and follower of these concepts, and package them in a beautiful, four-color format. The recipes contained within are appropriate for your blood type and compliant with the food lists, and they are delicious and made with love—love of food, love of health, and love of sharing this with others on both Kristin's and my part.

I invite you to join us on the continued journey of personalized living. I am confident that you will find a trusted companion in these cookbooks, and one who will make your life richer and healthier as you experiment with the recipes that were developed specifically to be right for your type.

IN THE BLOOD-TYPE world, B stands for Balance. To be as healthy as possible, Type B should not only strive for balance in their meals, but also in life. As Type As achieve health through a mostly vegetarian diet and Type O should maintain a protein-rich, carnivorous diet, Type B works best by enjoying the best of both worlds. Whereas with the other blood types there are large groups of foods to avoid, Type B has highly *Beneficial* foods in every category: meats, grains, dairy, fruits, and vegetables. Type B has a wide array of cheeses to select from, not to mention three *Neutrals* that are on most blood types' *Avoid* list: beer, red wine, and coffee . . . lucky you. Of course, *Neutrals* are not going to improve your health, but in moderation they won't harm you either. Let's briefly review what it means to be a Type B.

When structuring meals for the day, Type Bs should try to have a protein, complex carbohydrate, and vegetable with each dish. Protein is best achieved through red meats such as lamb, mutton, and rabbit as well as a variety of cheeses, beans, and an abundant selection of seafood. Chicken, shellfish, and soy proteins should be avoided. Between the selection of *Beneficial* and *Neutral* grains, there is not much to avoid besides corn. You will have ample choice between many delicious grains, breads, and pastas. Fruits and vegetable options are also plentiful, just be sure to avoid tomatoes.

Type Bs are fortunate to be known for their strong immune systems, aiding in their ability to be adaptable to various dietary and environmental influences. It's for this reason that Type Bs should eat a diverse and balanced diet. Disease susceptibility in Type B occurs when there are imbalances in the body, typically resulting in autoimmune disease or rare, slow-growing viruses. Type Bs are also at risk for Type I diabetes and chronic fatigue syndrome. Maintaining a balanced diet and adhering to Type B *Beneficials*, however, will help prevent these medical risks.

The Blood Type Diet has taken personalized nutrition to a higher level with the introduction of the influence Secretor Status has on our health.

Approximately 80 percent of the population are Secretors, which means that the majority of us secrete our blood-type antigens in our bodily fluids such as saliva and mucus. As I wrote in *Live Right 4 Your Type*:

> Subtyping your blood, especially your Secretor Status, provides an even greater specificity of identification. Your blood type doesn't just sit inert in your body. It is expressed in countless ways . . . A simple analogy would be a faucet. Depending on the water pressure, the faucet might pour or dribble . . . In the same way, your Secretor Status relates to how much and where your blood type antigen is expressed in your body.

Being a Secretor means that we can immediately attack viruses, bacteria, and other foreign bodies as they come in contact with our bodies, through secretions in our saliva. Non-Secretors do not have this first line of defense; however, their internal defenses are more powerful than Secretors. All of this means that some foods that are suitable for Secretors may not be for Non-Secretors (NS), and vice versa. To address this, we have tagged all recipes in this book that are appropriate for Non-Secretors, and when possible, substitutions are provided to make the other recipes acceptable and healthful for Non-Secretors.

Just as your food should be balanced, so should your exercise regimen. The most effective workout strategies for your blood type are those that balance moderate physical exertion with a mental component, so stick to hiking, biking, tennis, and swimming, most of which are also gentle on the knees.

In this book, you will find recipes, menus, and tools specifically designed for your Type B diet and Secretor Status. For more information, see *Eat Right 4 Your Type*, the *Blood Type B Food, Beverage and Supplement Lists,* or refer to your SWAMI© Personalized Nutrition Software Program guide if you have one (SWAMI is a proprietary software program designed to produce a unique, one-of-a-kind diet protocol based on your blood type, a series of biometric measurements and your personal history. See page 236 in the Appendix).

Type B is the adventurous blood type, encouraged to explore and try new things. Type B has the luxury of eating all kinds of interesting foods and eating them in combination with one another, so don't be afraid to dig in and get started on your own blood-type adventure.

First Things First

Beneficial Foods

Here is a list of basics to keep in your kitchen with the thought that there will be times when meals have to be spontaneous. If you have essentials from your *Beneficial* and *Neutral* lists on hand, no matter what you make, it will be something good for you.

Let's Start with the Fridge
Salad Base

Pick your favorite greens or mix it up each time you go to the grocery store, keeping these salad-base options in mind:

BENEFICIALS
  Cabbage
  Kale

NEUTRALS
Arugula	Escarole	Spinach
Boston Bibb	Red-leaf lettuce	

These will give you a great start to a last-minute salad or an added crunch to a sandwich.

Roasted Vegetables

The best thing you could do for yourself is to keep hearty fresh vegetables on hand. They are perfect to roast for dinner, make in bulk to add to your last-minute salad the next day, or throw in a frittata for breakfast. Roasted vegetables are a terrific leftover to keep on hand. Most vegetables work well when tossed with olive oil, sea salt, and roasted in a 375-degree oven for 12 to 20 minutes (depending on the size and density of the vegetables.) Here are a few that are both *Beneficial* to Type B and take well to roasting:

BENEFICIALS

Beets	Kale
Broccoli	Parsnips
Carrots	Peppers
Cauliflower	Sweet potatoes/yams
Eggplant	Turnips

NEUTRALS

Asparagus	Potatoes
Celeriac	Squash
Fennel	Zucchini
Onions	

Keeping a few of these vegetables in your fridge each week will come in handy and is a perfect way to add more *Beneficials* to your diet.

Fruit

Most people don't have a problem incorporating fruit in their diet. It is a perfect snack, paired with nuts or nut butters, used to make desserts, and added to cereal or salads. Some fruits even work well in savory dishes. Below is a list of *Beneficial* fruit for Type B:

BENEFICIALS

Bananas	Pineapples
Cranberries	Plums
Grapes	Watermelon
Papayas	

Milk

Type Bs are among the few who benefit from cow's milk, which is a great source of protein. The best milk options for Type Bs are:

Nonfat or 2 percent cow's milk

 Type B

Protein

The Type B diet is based on balanced protein and vegetable consumption, so it is important to keep a diverse supply of proteins to accompany vegetables and grains at each meal. We suggest keeping two fresh types of proteins in the fridge and then two to three in the freezer for backup. Prepare more meat than you need and save the rest as leftovers to enjoy the next day for lunch or to add to a casserole. Here are a few staples that are useful to have on hand. Please note, it is recommended that all poultry be organic and all beef be grass-fed and organic.

BENEFICIALS

Cheeses (cottage cheese, farmer cheese, feta, goat cheese, kefir, mozzarella, ricotta)

Lamb (cheaper and contain more lean meat than chops or rack)

Nut butter (walnut butter made from black walnuts)

Seafood (cod, flounder, grouper, halibut, mahimahi, salmon, sole)

NEUTRALS

Beef tips

Cheeses (Brie, Camembert, Cheddar, Colby, cream cheese, Gouda, Gruyere, Jarlsberg, Monterey Jack, Muenster, Parmesan, provolone, Swiss)

Eggs

Ground beef (90 percent lean or leaner)

Nut butters (almond, pecan, or macadamia. Almond butter is inexpensive and easily found in supermarkets or natural food stores.)

Seafood (catfish, herring, orange roughy, red snapper, sole, squid, tilapia, whitefish)

Turkey tenderloins

Filling up Your Freezer

Smoothies

Making smoothies is a great alternative for breakfast or a perfect protein-filled snack. They are a go-to recipe that you should be sure you have ingredients for at all times. Of course, fresh fruit can be used when in season. Mix in some frozen fruits and vegetables into the smoothie for a thicker consistency, however. Here are a few *Beneficial* options:

BENEFICIALS

Bananas

Kale

Pineapple

Figs	Peaches	Strawberries
Mangos	Raspberries	

Leftovers

It's always helpful to double the recipe when making foods that freeze easily such as:

Chili	Lasagna	Sauces
Cookies	Muffins	Stews
Crackers	Pesto	

Type B 11

Pesto can be stored in BPA-free ice cube trays for individual servings. On the following pages, you will find more information on safe food storage as well as suggestions for cooking in bulk.

Protein

Just like keeping fresh protein options in your fridge, it is always helpful to keep at least a few in the freezer as well. To defrost meats, poultry, or seafood, take them out the day before and put them in the refrigerator. It is recommended that all beef be grass fed and organic.

BENEFICIALS

Beef tips
Ground beef (90 percent lean or leaner)
Lamb steaks (cheaper and contain more lean meat than chops or rack)
Turkey (ground, tenderloins, whole)
Seafood (cod, flounder, grouper, halibut, mahimahi, salmon, sole)

NEUTRALS

Seafood (catfish, herring, orange roughy, red snapper, scallops, squid, tilapia, whitefish)

Time to Get in That Pantry
Snacks

The first thing we all go into the pantry for is to grab a quick bite on the run or pack a snack to ship off to school with the kids. It's pretty important that these midday treats are balanced and wholesome; the best way to make that happen is to stock that pantry right. Here are a few staples for Type Bs:

Almond butter
Brown rice cakes
Dark chocolate (70 percent or higher)
Dried fruit (banana chips, cranberries, figs, prunes)
Fresh fruit (bananas, grapes, papaya, pineapple, plums, watermelon)
Nuts (almonds, pecans, macadamia nuts, walnuts)
Spelt crackers
Whole-grain cereals (made from oat, spelt, or brown rice)

If you want to prep ahead for those times when you are in a rush, mix combinations of nuts, dried fruit, and maybe even a little dark chocolate, and divide into single servings. Store in small glass sealable containers and take them in the car, on the plane, or anywhere you are headed.

Drinks

Drinking water is always the best option, but when you want to add a little flavor to your beverage repertoire, dabble in these *Beneficial* teas or *Neutral* drinks, but try not to go overboard with *Neutrals*. There are a few drink recipes in this book.

BENEFICIALS

   Grape juice
   Pineappale juice
   Teas (ginger, green, licorice, peppermint, rose hip)

NEUTRALS

   Beer   Coffee
   Black tea   Red wine

Grains/Legumes

Grains should be an integral part of the Type B diet, eaten in balance with protein and vegetables at each meal. There are quite a few grains to choose from, which are both *Beneficial* and *Neutral* and will add variety to any meal. Quinoa, for example, cooks in 12 minutes and is a light but filling side for a fast weeknight dinner. Beans are also a perfect way to add satiating proteins and carbohydrates to salads, casseroles, stews, dips, and soups.

    Beans (kidney, lima, navy)
    Whole grains (millet, oat bran, oat meal, puffed rice, rice bran, rice
       cakes, spelt)

Seasonings

Making healthy food taste good is non-negotiable. One quick trick to doing so is by knowing your way around your spice cabinet. Herbs and spices are calorie free and flavor packed. The spices listed below also happen to be terrific for your Type B body. Keep a jar of homemade bread crumbs on hand for a quick topping on a casserole, used as turkey breading, or to bread seafood. Additionally, as much as we would like to repress our sweet tooth, it is an unrealistic expectation for most, so stock up on natural sweeteners like agave and maple syrup, although try to use sparingly.

BENEFICIALS

    Basic Bread Crumbs **NS**
    Olive oil
    Molasses
    Spices (cayenne pepper, curry, ginger, horseradish, parsley)

NEUTRALS

    Spices (anise, basil, bay leaf, caraway, cardamom, carob, chili pow-
       der, chive, clove, coriander, cumin, garlic, marjoram, mustard,
       nutmeg, oregano, paprika, red pepper flakes, peppermint, sage,
       tamari, tamarind, tarragon, thyme, turmeric, vanilla)
    Maple syrup
    Agave nectar
    Vinegar

Recipe Ideas for Last-Minute Cooking

Time-Saving Tricks

Make these recipes in bulk and store in your freezer to grab on the go: flax chips, smoothies in individual portions, baked goods, chili, granola, soups, casseroles, pesto in ice-cube trays, or stews.

When making dressings or condiments, double or triple the recipe and store it in the refrigerator for future use. If you are making a recipe that uses one lemon, you might as well do it with three and save yourself the prep and clean-up again and again.

Utilize Roasted Vegetables

Let's reemphasize here how amazingly useful leftover roasted vegetables can be. Not only are they ready to be thrown into just about any savory dish, but they add tremendous flavor with no effort whatsoever. Here are a few examples where you can toss in roasted vegetables and have a tasty new dish:

Casseroles	Omelets	Soufflés
Cold pasta salad	Pizza	Spring rolls
Crêpes	Quiches	Taco salads
Frittata	Rice	Vegetable tarts
Lettuce wraps	Salads	

Next time you make roasted vegetables for dinner, do yourself a favor and double up on that recipe.

Review Your Stock

Now that you have the basics, it's time to take a look at some of the *Avoids*. You have lived your whole life eating whatever you want. Now you open your cabinets and think, how do I start over? but the answer is simple: you don't have to. You just have to emphasize the healthy choices that you are now privy to. You should ditch anything that is categorized *Best Avoided* for your type; listed below are a few places where *Avoids* may be lurking and ready to sabotage your otherwise perfect, new diet.

- Open up the fridge—take inventory of all condiments, sauces, stocks, and other processed foods.
- Open the pantry—familiarize yourself with the ingredients in your snacks, cereals, pastas, spices, and other foods.
- Open the freezer—remove frozen dinners. Just do it. You can be sure they are not doing you any good. Other than that, the same applies here as above: evaluate what you have, and review ingredients just to get yourself acquainted with what you are dealing with.

Once you have done that, take out all questionable subjects and line them up on the counter or table. Refer to the Type B diet in *Eat Right 4 Your Type*, the *Blood Type B Food, Beverage, and Supplement List*, or refer to your SWAMI personalized nutrition report food lists. Check out your *Avoids*, as this will be the most efficient way of eliminating those foods that are best *Avoided*.

Please note that *Avoids* are not limited to the examples listed below. Here is a rundown of the main offenders:

Corn

Corn has become a hot topic in the food world. The movie *Food Inc.* helped explain to many people that the mass production of corn has become a national, if not global, issue. With the introduction of genetically modified organisms (GMOs) or foods that are genetically altered to optimize their growing potential, corn quite literally became another species. As an *Avoid* for Type B, eliminating corn gives us yet another opportunity to clean our diet. Due to our society's dependence on corn, it is used in a wide range of processed goods, making it virtually impossible to avoid altogether.

We will do our best to outline where corn is generally hidden, but know, too, that with this diet, it is ok to run into an *Avoid* once in a while without sabotaging your progress. If you are not acutely sick and are simply using the Blood Type Diet for general health, you only have to be 80 percent compliant to see 100 percent results. How forgiving is that?

The following are a few places corn exists:

Alcohol (some)
Artificial flavorings
Artificial sweeteners
Ascorbic acid
Aspartame
Baked goods (some)
Baking powder (some)
Canned fruits and some
    vegetables
Caramel color
Cereal
Cheese spreads
Citric acid
Confectioners' sugar
Corn flour
Corn starch
Corn syrup
Food starch
Grits
Hominy
Hydrolyzed vegetable protein
Ice cream (some)
Instant coffee/teas

Ketchup
Licorice
Maize
Malt/malt syrup
Modified food starch
Molasses (some)
Polenta
Popcorn
Prepared mustard (some)
Salad dressings
Salt (iodized)
Soda
Splenda
Sucrose
Sugar (if not cane or beet)
Sweet beverages (containing
    corn syrup)
Taco shells
Tomato sauce (with corn syrup)
Vitamins (some)
Xanthan gum
Yeast (some)
Yogurt (with corn syrup)

Soy

When most people hear they have to avoid soy, they say, "No problem, I can't stand tofu anyway." Unfortunately, soy is not only found in obvious places like soy sauce, tofu, or soy cheese. Due to its perceived adaptability, soy is used as a blank canvas to adapt to any flavor or texture. It is relatively inexpensive to produce, and it can be found in almost all processed foods today. The good news is, avoiding soy means avoiding most packaged foods that probably contain many ingredients that are unhealthy for you, so try to think of it as a great reminder to eat whole, pure foods as often as possible. Below is a list of foods that generally contain soy or are soy-based products. It is important to read food labels to make sure you are totally avoiding soy.

Artificial or natural flavors	Soy milk
Canned tuna (some)	Soy oil
Chocolate	Soy sauce
Crisco	Store-bought baked goods
Edamame	(some)
Fermented bean paste	Store-bought broth (some)
Gravy (some)	Soups (some)
Hydrolyzed vegetable protein	Spice blends (some)
Mayonnaise	Tamari
Miso	Tempeh
Mono-diglyceride	Teriyaki sauce
Monosodium glutamate	Textured vegetable protein
Salad dressings	Tofu
Soy cheese	Whipped toppings
Soy flour	Worcestershire sauce

Wheat

Although Type Bs do not have to be gluten-free, it is beneficial for you to be as wheat free as possible, both for optimal weight loss and health. Luckily for you, there are plenty of non-wheat options to cook with and to buy as healthier substitutions. Spelt or brown rice breads are readily available in health food stores and online, and they are very close to the texture and taste of wheat breads.

Here are a few places where wheat exists:

Baking powder (some)
Beer
Blue cheese (some)
Bread crumbs
Breaded fish
Breads
Brewer's yeast
Broth (some)
Bulgur
Candies (some)
Caramel color (some)
Cereal
Chewing gum
Cold cuts (some)
Cookies
Cornbread
Couscous
Crackers
Croutons
Dumplings
Farina
Flavored extracts (some)
Food starch or modified food
    starch (some)
Graham flour
Gravy
Hot dogs
Hush puppies
Hydrolyzed plant protein
Hydrolyzed vegetable protein
Ice cream (some)
Kamut
Malt (flavoring, and vinegar)
Matzo
Meat loaf
Meatballs
"Natural flavor" (either soy
    or gluten)
Pancakes
Pasta (including orzo)
Pastries
Pie crust
Pita bread
Pizza crust
Potato chips (some)
Pretzels
Salad dressings
Seitan
Semolina
Soups
Soy sauce
Spice mixtures (some)
Syrup
Tamari
Teriyaki sauce
Textured vegetable protein
Waffles
Wheat
Wheat protein
Wheatgrass
Worcestershire sauce

Chicken

Chicken seems to be the most difficult exclusion for Type Bs. The most challenging part of no longer eating chicken is figuring out options when eating out, because in your own kitchen it can easily be replaced with turkey in most recipes. Because Type Bs are made to have balanced diets, however, you can see that there are many options still available when dining out.

The Rest

Other than corn, soy, wheat, and chicken, it will be straightforward to determine what else to take out of your cabinets, fridge, and freezer. Take the time to go through your list of *Avoid*s and remove them from your house. If you have canned goods, and nonperishables, you can donate to your local food bank. To find a food bank in your area, go to http://feed ingamerica.org.

You should be all cleared out now, so you are ready to go to the store and grab a few essentials to fill in the gaps.

How to Read These Recipes

This cookbook is designed to be as practical and helpful to the Blood Type dieter as possible. We took into consideration that many families could be cooking for multiple blood types or preparing meals for friends with varying blood types. In order to make doing so practical, each of the *Eat Right 4 Your Type Personalized Cookbooks* contains the same or similar recipe ideas with different executions to suit the needs of each blood type. You will find the recipe titles almost identical in each book; however, ingredients and methods might vary quite a bit. There are many recipes that are *Beneficial* across the board and are marked with an (A/B/AB/O) to identify that they are universal to every type. For example, every blood type has a pancake recipe; however, Type Bs have *Beneficial* grains that might be on the *Avoid* list for other types, so each recipe contains different flours.

Every recipe is also written to contain as many *Beneficial* foods as possible with the understanding that taste is still of the utmost importance. After all, you are not going to be inclined to dive into a kale cookie, but you won't be able to resist Pasta Carbonara with Crispy Kale. The point is that we want you coming back for more each time to see that eating right for your blood type is as far from sacrifice as is indulging in a bar of chocolate.

As you make your way through this book, you will notice that once in a while there is a highlighted section called "Featured Ingredient." There are several ingredients used in this book that you may not have come across before, some that are *Beneficial* for your diet and some that are *Beneficial* for your taste buds. In an effort to familiarize you with these ingredients, there is a brief summary explaining a little about what that ingredient is, and how or why it is used. Don't be afraid to experiment with unfamiliar territory.

Many people who follow the Blood Type Diet come to my office or have used the tests on my website (www.dadamo.com) to create a specific diet plan for themselves. If you have done that, you have a SWAMI personalized nutrition report that may vary slightly from the general Type B diet because it takes into consideration family and medical history, Secretor Status, and GenoType. (The GenoType is a further refinement of my work in personalized nutrition. It uses a variety of simple measurements, combined with blood type data, to classify individuals as one of six basic Epigenotypes: The Hunter, Gatherer, Teacher, Explorer, Warrior, and Nomad types.). Due to the variations in *Beneficial*, *Neutral*, and *Best Avoided* foods, there may be some recipes containing ingredients that do not suit you as an individual. Please do not skip these recipes entirely. There is always a way to make quick and easy substitutions. (See "Useful Tools: Substitutions," page 215.) As a quick piece of advice, however, vegetables can be easily swapped out—leafy greens for other leafy greens, a specific type of beans for another, or in some cases, simply omitted from the recipe if they are not a star component.

You will see that recipes are also tagged according to Secretor Status. Some recipes are not appropriate for Non-Secretors, but are fine for Secretors (see recipe legend below) in most instances. When this is the case, there are simple substitutions to adapt the recipe for Non-Secretors. In a few cases, however, the recipe will be an *Avoid* altogether for a Type B Non-Secretor.

In many of the recipes in this book, you will see sea salt written as "sea salt, to taste," and might be wondering what that means or how much to add. Salt can make or break your dish, but if you add too much, there is no going back. Try adding a little at a time, taste, and add more if needed. What is *a little*? Well, start with pinching a bit between your fingers and sprinkling it into your dish, give it a minute to incorporate, and then taste. If you were to measure a pinch, it would be a little less than ⅛ of a teaspoon.

Remember to read each recipe in its entirety before starting to ensure you know how much time it will take and if there are any ingredients you will need to buy ahead of time. Finally, enjoy making, eating, and sharing these recipes.

RECIPE LEGEND:
- An * is used when a recipe ingredient needs further instruction, substitution, or comment. This information is found at the bottom of a recipe.
- All recipes are appropriate for Type B Secretors.

- **NS** represents a recipe that is appropriate for Type B Non-Secretors.
- Recipe ingredients that are NOT appropriate for Type B Non-Secretors **NS** are notated with appropriate acceptable substitutions within recipe ingredients.

A REVIEW OF THE FOOD LISTS:

Throughout this book we refer to a number of places to find the comprehensive foods lists for the Blood Type Diet. Here's a recap of where you can find the lists so you can use the one that is right for you:

- *Eat Right 4 Your Type,* which provides the entry point into the Blood Type Diet
- *Live Right 4 Your Type*, which incorporates the value of the Secretor Status
- *Blood Type B Food, Beverage, and Supplement Lists from Eat Right 4 Your Type*, a handy pocket guide with the basic food lists
- *Change Your Genetic Destiny* (originally published as *The Geno-Type Diet*, which provides a further refinement of the diet by using blood type, secretor status, and a series of biometric measurements to further individualize your food lists)
- SWAMI Personalized Nutrition Software, designed to harness the power of computers and artificial intelligence, using their tremendous precision and speed to help tailor unique, one-of-a-kind diets. From its extensive knowledge base, SWAMI can evaluate more than 700 foods for more than 200 individual attributes (such as cholesterol level, gluten content, presence of antioxidants, etc.) to determine if that food is either a superfood or toxin for you. It provides a specific, unique diet in an easy-to-read, user-friendly format, complete with food lists, recipes, and meal planning.

Breakfast

Breakfast recipes were written with diversity in mind, so that you do not end up eating the same thing every day. The idea here is to alternate: one day eggs, the next quinoa or granola, and so on, in order to keep providing your body with different nutrients each day. You will probably notice that the biggest change in these recipes is the types of flour used. Don't be intimidated; try one simple recipe like pancakes to get your feet wet and move on to the rest. Once you have the new flour on hand, the rest is just like any other recipe.

Quinoa Muesli

½ cup quinoa

½ cup water

½ cup 2 percent cow's milk

¼ teaspoon sea salt

2 tablespoons dried cherries

1 tablespoon dried cranberries

2 tablespoons slivered almonds

2 tablespoons chopped walnuts

2 teaspoons maple syrup

¼ cup crunchy rice cereal

1. Rinse quinoa. Combine in a small saucepan with water, milk, salt, cherries, and cranberries, and bring to a boil. Cook 10 minutes, turn off the heat, and let sit an additional 4 to 5 minutes. Quinoa will absorb all the water and become light and fluffy when done.

2. While the quinoa cooks, toast almonds and walnuts in a dry skillet for about 2 minutes or until slightly golden brown. Watch nuts carefully; because of their high fat content, they have a tendency to burn easily.

3. Fluff cooked quinoa with a fork and add toasted nuts and maple syrup. Top with crunchy rice cereal and add more milk if desired.

4. Serve immediately.

▶ SERVES 2

featured ingredient

quinoa/quinoa flour

Quinoa, an ancient grain cultivated by the Incan tribes, has only recently become popular again. It is a fantastic meal in itself because it is high in fiber and contains all nine amino acids, making it a complete protein source. When cooked, quinoa has a slightly nutty flavor and a light, soft texture with a subtle crunch from the outer shell of the grain. It can be used in most recipes where rice is called for, and can even be eaten with dried fruit and nuts for a warm breakfast treat. Quinoa is also ground into flour for use in breads, pancakes, and many baked goods.

4 cups crispy rice cereal

1 cup chopped walnuts

1 cup chopped pecans

¼ cup halved whole flaxseeds

¼ cup blackstrap molasses

2 teaspoons olive oil

1 tablespoon agave

⅛ teaspoon sea salt

¼ cup water

1 cup halved dried cherries

½ cup dried cranberries

1. Preheat oven to 350 degrees. Line a sheet pan with parchment paper and set aside.

2. In a large bowl, combine rice cereal, walnuts, pecans, and flax-seeds. Set aside.

3. In a small saucepan, warm molasses, olive oil, agave, and salt with water over medium heat for about 2 minutes, whisking to combine.

4. Pour molasses mixture over granola mixture, toss to coat, and spread onto prepared sheet pan. Bake 10 minutes. Reduce oven temperature to 300 degrees.

5. Take granola out of the oven, toss, and place back in the oven. Bake an additional 25 minutes.

6. Toss with cherries and cranberries.

7. Serve warm or cool fully, and store in an airtight, glass container for up to 2 weeks or in the freezer for up to 2 months.

▶ MAKES 32 (½-CUP) SERVINGS

Nut Butter–Granola Boats NS

3 tablespoons walnut or almond butter

⅓ cup granola*

Sea salt, to taste

2 bananas

1. Stir nut butter, granola, and salt until granola is evenly coated.

2. Peel bananas, and slice in half down the center and then in half lengthwise, so you have 4 long pieces of banana. Spoon 2 teaspoons granola mixture on each piece of banana and enjoy.

*See Blackstrap-Cherry Rice Granola NS recipe (page 25).

▶ SERVES 2

egg salad:

2 teaspoons olive oil

½ cup cooked or canned kidney beans, drained and rinsed

3 hardboiled eggs

¼ cup mozzarella cheese

1 tablespoon chopped parsley

2 cups mixed baby greens

Sea salt, to taste

dressing:

½ teaspoon mustard powder

1 tablespoon olive oil

1 tablespoon lemon juice

1 tablespoon onion, grated

Sea salt, to taste

1. In a small skillet, heat olive oil over medium heat. Toast kidney beans 2 to 3 minutes until warm and slightly crunchy. Set aside.

2. Remove eggs from shells, and use a fork to break apart in a bowl. Set aside. In a separate bowl, whisk together all dressing ingredients. Pour over eggs and toss.

3. Add beans, cheese, and parsley to eggs, and toss. Serve over mixed baby greens.

▶ SERVES 4

1. Heat a large skillet over medium heat, and coat with nonstick cooking spray.

2. Add bacon and cook 3 to 4 minutes, flip, and cook an additional 2 to 3 minutes on the opposite side for crispy bacon. Remove from pan, let cool, then crumble and set aside.

3. Whisk eggs and egg whites in a small bowl. Set aside. In the same skillet, add olive oil and reduce heat slightly. Add spinach, sauté 2 minutes, and season mixture with sea salt to taste. Pour eggs over spinach, cooking gently until done, about 2 minutes. Turn off heat and add reserved bacon and cheese.

4. Spoon mixture on toast and serve immediately.

▶ SERVES 4

Nonstick cooking spray
3 strips turkey bacon
3 large whole eggs
3 large egg whites
2 teaspoons olive oil
2 cups fresh spinach
Sea salt, to taste
¼ cup mozzarella cheese
4 slices brown rice/millet or spelt toast

tip: If the bacon is not as crispy as you like, you can add a drizzle of olive oil to help it along.

featured ingredient

turkey bacon (nitrate- /preservative-free)

Not all turkey bacon is the same. There are many types and brands on the market, but most are artificially derived, and loaded with salt, preservatives, and full of nitrates . . . all things you absolutely do not want to be eating. There are a few companies that make turkey bacon without these unhealthy and artificial additives; they can be found at your local natural foods store and in some mainstream grocery stores.

Swiss Chard and Cremini Frittata NS

2 teaspoons ghee

¼ cup finely diced Spanish onion

1 cup diced cremini mushrooms

3 cups chopped Swiss chard

3 large whole eggs

3 large egg whites

2 tablespoons spelt flour

Sea salt, to taste

1 teaspoon chopped fresh tarragon

1 teaspoon olive oil

1. Preheat oven to 375 degrees.

2. Melt ghee in an ovenproof sauté pan over medium heat. Sauté onion, mushrooms, and Swiss chard for 4 to 5 minutes, until chard has wilted and vegetables are tender. Set aside.

3. While onion mixture is cooking, whisk together eggs, egg whites, flour, salt, and tarragon in a large bowl. Add olive oil to skillet and pour egg mixture over vegetables. Cook for about 1 minute, just until set.

4. Transfer pan to oven and bake 6 to 8 minutes, or until firm and edges are golden.

▶ SERVES 4

Broccoli-Feta Frittata NS

1 head broccoli

¼ teaspoon sea salt

1 tablespoon plus 2 teaspoons olive oil, divided

3 large whole eggs

2 large egg whites

⅓ cup crumbled feta

½ cup chopped spinach

¼ cup finely diced chives

2 teaspoon brown rice or spelt flour

1 tablespoon chopped oregano

1. Preheat oven to 375 degrees.

2. Dice broccoli into bite-size pieces, place in a single layer on a baking sheet, and sprinkle with a dash of sea salt and 1 tablespoon olive oil. Bake 15 minutes.

3. In a medium-size bowl, whisk eggs, egg whites, feta, spinach, chives, flour, oregano, and salt until well combined.

4. Brush a medium-size, ovenproof skillet with remaining 2 teaspoons olive oil and heat over medium heat, to create a nonstick surface. Add egg mixture to hot pan with broccoli. Cook 1 to 2 minutes, lifting the side of the eggs gently with your spatula to encourage uncooked egg to run down into the bottom of the skillet.

5. If the handle of your skillet is rubber, wrap tightly with tinfoil to prevent melting. Place skillet under the broiler for 2 minutes, or until the eggs set and brown very slightly on the edges.

6. Serve warm.

▶ SERVES 4

Maple-Sausage Scramble (NS)

¼ cup finely chopped white onion

3 cups chopped kale

1 cup diced zucchini

⅓ cup finely diced red bell peppers

4 teaspoons olive oil, divided

½ pound ground turkey sausage

1 tablespoon maple syrup

3 large eggs

2 large egg whites

1 tablespoon water

Large-grain sea salt, to taste

¼ cup diced kefir cheese

1. In a large skillet, sauté onion, kale, zucchini, and peppers in 2 teaspoons olive oil over medium heat for 3 to 4 minutes, or until vegetables are aromatic and tender and kale is bright green and wilted. Remove from skillet and set aside.

2. Brown turkey sausage in the same skillet with remaining 2 teaspoons olive oil over medium heat, breaking into bite-size pieces until cooked through, about 5 to 6 minutes. Drizzle with maple syrup, and stir to coat. Add sausage to vegetables and set aside.

3. Return skillet to stovetop and reduce heat to medium-low. Whisk eggs and egg whites with water and salt to taste, and add to skillet. Stir gently with a heat-safe spatula until firm and cooked through. Add sausage and vegetables to the skillet, and stir to combine.

4. Serve topped with kefir cheese.

▶ SERVES 4

EAT RIGHT FOR YOUR TYPE PERSONALIZED COOKBOOK

1. In a large sauté pan, heat olive oil over medium heat. Add onions and fennel, and sauté 3 to 4 minutes, or until tender. Remove from heat and let cool to room temperature, about 10 minutes.

2. Place ground turkey in a large bowl, and add fennel seed, paprika, salt, chili powder, garlic, pear, maple syrup, and cooled vegetables. Use your hands to incorporate all ingredients into the meat, but do not over mix.

3. Form meat into small, hot dog–shaped links. Cook 8 to 10 minutes or until meat is browned on all sides and inside of the sausage is no longer pink.

4. Serve warm alone or alongside scrambled eggs for a protein-packed breakfast.

▶ SERVES 4

2 teaspoons olive oil

½ cup finely diced onion

½ cup finely diced fennel

1 pound ground turkey meat

1 teaspoon fennel seed

1 teaspoon paprika

1 teaspoon sea salt

¼ teaspoon chili powder

1 clove garlic, minced

½ cup finely diced Bosc pear

2 teaspoons maple syrup

Savory Herb and Cheese Bread Pudding NS

2 teaspoons olive oil, plus more for greasing

1 teaspoon ghee

2 cups diced onion

2 cups quartered white mushrooms

2 cups diced zucchini

6 cups torn kale

Sea salt, to taste

8 cups (1-inch) bread cubes (sprouted wheat or spelt bread)

1 cup 2 percent cow's milk

1 cup Vegetable Stock*

4 large eggs, beaten

1 teaspoon fresh thyme

1 teaspoon fresh rosemary

1 teaspoon fresh sage

1 cup mozzarella cheese

1. Preheat oven to 350 degrees. Grease a 9" x 11" baking dish with olive oil and set aside.

2. In a large skillet, heat ghee and 2 teaspoons olive oil over medium heat. Sauté onion, mushrooms, zucchini, and kale until tender, about 5 to 6 minutes. Season with salt, and set aside.

3. Spread bread cubes in a single layer on a baking sheet. Toast for 3 to 4 minutes, until slightly golden brown. Toss in a large bowl with vegetables.

4. Whisk together milk, stock, eggs, thyme, rosemary, and sage. Pour over bread and vegetables, and toss to combine. Pour the entire mixture into the prepared baking dish. Top with mozzarella cheese and bake, covered, for 35 minutes. Uncover, and bake an additional 10 minutes, until cheese is bubbling and slightly browned.

5. Serve warm.

*See Vegetable Stock NS recipe (page 211).

▶ SERVES 12

1. Preheat oven to 350 degrees. Spray 4 (12-oz.) ramekins with nonstick cooking spray, place in a baking dish, and set aside.

2. In a saucepan over medium heat, melt ghee and whisk in flour. Gradually add milk and stock, whisking continuously until thickened, about 3 to 4 minutes. Once mixture is thick and resembles the consistency of yogurt, remove from the heat and let cool completely.

3. In a food processor, puree spinach and bell pepper. Place pureed vegetables onto cheesecloth or paper towels, wrap the cloth around the vegetables, and strain excess liquid by gently squeezing the vegetable juice through the cloth. Place vegetables in a bowl, and whisk in egg yolks, basil, cheese, cayenne, and salt. Set aside.

4. Fold milk mixture into vegetable mixture and set aside.

5. In a dry, glass bowl, beat egg whites with a hand mixer until they form stiff peaks. Fold the egg whites, one-third at a time, into the vegetables. Spoon mixture into prepared ramekins, and fill the baking dish halfway with hot water. Carefully place in the oven and bake for 45 minutes or until tester inserted into ramekin comes out clean.

6. Serve immediately.

*See Vegetable Stock **NS** recipe (page 211).

▶ SERVES 4

Spinach-Pepper Soufflé **NS**

1 tablespoon ghee

2 tablespoons spelt or oat flour

½ cup 2 percent cow's milk

½ cup Vegetable Stock*

2 cups packed spinach

1 cup chopped red bell pepper

2 large egg yolks

¼ cup chopped basil

¼ cup grated Gruyere cheese

¼ teaspoon cayenne pepper

Sea salt, to taste

4 egg whites, at room temperature

featured ingredient

spelt flour

Spelt is an ancient grain related to wheat, with a slightly nuttier flavor and a greater amount of nutrients. It can be used as a direct substitution in almost any recipe calling for wheat flour. (Although spelt does contain gluten, it does not seem to be a problem for people who cannot tolerate wheat.) Spelt can be purchased in a variety of forms, from the whole grain to flour, pasta, and bread. Store spelt in the refrigerator, to retain the maximum benefits of its nutritional value.

Oat Crêpes

⅓ cup oat flour

⅓ cup spelt flour

¼ teaspoon sea salt

1¼ cups 2 percent cow's milk

2 large eggs

1 tablespoon plus 1 teaspoon melted ghee or butter, divided

1. In a medium bowl, whisk flours and sea salt.

2. Combine milk, eggs, and 1 tablespoon melted ghee, and beat well. Add to flour mixture, and whisk until well blended. Cover and place in the refrigerator for 1 hour.

3. Heat a large sauté pan over medium heat. When the pan is hot, add remaining 1 teaspoon ghee and brush evenly across the bottom of the pan. Using a ¼-cup measuring cup, scoop batter into pan and quickly turn the pan in circular motions to spread the batter into a very thin layer. Let cook 1 minute or until the batter firms and edges lift slightly off the pan. Use an offset spatula to flip and cook 1 additional minute.

▶ SERVES 4

tip: For an indulgent treat, top with banana slices, walnuts, and Chocolate Syrup NS (page 209).

EAT RIGHT FOR YOUR TYPE PERSONALIZED COOKBOOK

muffins:

2 cups spelt flour

1 cup oat flour

2 teaspoons baking powder

½ teaspoon baking soda

½ teaspoon fine-grain sea salt

⅛ teaspoon ground cloves

½ teaspoon ground ginger

¼ teaspoon allspice (**NS** omit allspice and add ¼ teaspoon nutmeg)

1 (15-oz.) can organic sweet potatoes

½ cup honey

2 large eggs

½ cup 2 percent cow's milk

topping:

¼ cup rolled oats

⅓ cup finely chopped pecans

1 tablespoon honey

1 tablespoon almond or light olive oil

¼ cup Carob Extract™*

1. Preheat oven to 350 degrees. Line a 12-cup muffin tin with paper liners and set aside.

2. In a large bowl, stir together flours, baking powder, baking soda, salt, cloves, ginger, and allspice until well combined.

3. In a separate bowl, whisk sweet potatoes, honey, eggs, and milk. Add the sweet potato mixture to the flour mixture and stir to incorporate. Divide batter evenly among prepared muffin tins.

4. Combine topping ingredients in a bowl and toss with a fork. Sprinkle topping evenly on each muffin and drizzle with Carob Extract™.

5. Bake 20 to 25 minutes, or until a cake tester inserted into muffin comes out clean.

*Information about purchasing Carob Extract™ can be found in Appendix II: Products (page 235).

▶ SERVES 12

1. Preheat waffle maker.

2. In a large bowl, whisk dry ingredients together until well combined.

3. In a separate bowl, whisk wet ingredients. Add wet ingredients to dry, and mix until free of lumps. Fold in cooked rice.

4. Spoon batter into waffle maker just to the rim, close, and cook according to settings on your waffle maker. Waffles should be firm with a slightly crunchy exterior and soft interior.

5. Serve warm.

▶ SERVES 4

1½ cups spelt flour

½ cup oat flour

2 tablespoons flaxseeds

½ teaspoon sea salt

2 teaspoons baking powder

2 large eggs

2 cups 2 percent cow's milk

2 tablespoons olive oil

2 tablespoons applesauce

1 cup cooked wild rice

featured ingredient

flaxseeds

Flaxseeds are small with a hard, smooth surface and are packed with omega-3 fatty acids as well as manganese, fiber, and other nutrients. Foods rich in omega-3s are a healthy addition to any diet and provide anti-inflammatory benefits for Type Bs, specifically in their ability to fight cancer and diabetes. Flaxseeds can be added to smoothies, baked goods, or even used as a topping on salads. When submerged in warm water, flaxseeds bind together with the water and form a gelatin that is helpful in gluten-free baking and, if drank, will help keep you "regular."

Blueberry-Macadamia Muffins

1. Preheat oven to 350 degrees. Line a 12-cup muffin tin with paper liners and set aside.

2. In a large bowl, combine dry ingredients. Set aside.

3. In a separate bowl, whisk wet ingredients to combine. Add the wet ingredients to the dry ingredients, stirring to combine. Fold in macadamia nuts and blueberries. Divide batter evenly among prepared muffin tins and bake for 25 to 28 minutes, or until a cake tester inserted into muffin comes out clean.

4. Let muffins cool before serving.

▶ SERVES 12

1½ cups spelt flour

1 cup oat flour

½ teaspoon salt

2 teaspoons baking powder

1 teaspoon baking soda

2 large eggs

½ cup agave

½ teaspoon lemon zest

3 tablespoons light olive oil

½ cup applesauce

½ cup plus 2 tablespoons 2 percent cow's milk

⅓ cup mashed banana (about ½ medium banana)

½ cup chopped macadamia nuts

1 cup organic (fresh or frozen) blueberries

1. Combine flours, baking powder, and salt.

2. In a separate bowl, whisk eggs, milk, and olive oil. Add to flour mixture and stir until well combined and free of lumps.

3. Spray a skillet with nonstick cooking spray and place over medium-low heat. Spoon ¼ cup batter into skillet at a time, and let cook 1 to 2 minutes per side.

4. Serve warm. (If making a large batch, keep pancakes in the oven at 200 degrees, draped with a slightly damp paper towel.)

▶ SERVES 4

¾ cup spelt flour

¼ cup oat flour

2 teaspoons baking powder

½ teaspoon fine-grain sea salt

2 large eggs

1 cup nonfat cow's milk

2 tablespoons olive oil

feature ingredient

oat flour

Oats have a delicious, creamy flavor, and add smooth texture to baked goods. You can make oat flour by grinding quick-cooking oats in your food processor until fine. Naturally rich in fiber, one benefit of including oats in your diet is their ability to satiate your appetite, so you will not feel hungry soon after your meal. Oat flour is not a self-rising flour because it doesn't contain gluten, so it's best to combine it with spelt or wheat when baking. This is why most of the recipes in this book call for a combination of oat and spelt flours.

Cherry Scones NS

scones:

½ cup dried cherries, halved

1 cup spelt flour, plus more for rolling

½ cup oat flour

¼ cup almond flour

2 teaspoons baking powder

½ teaspoon sea salt

4 tablespoons butter, chilled

¼ cup 2 percent cow's milk

1 large egg

1 teaspoon lemon zest

⅓ cup agave

topping:

2 tablespoons agave

2 tablespoons almond flour

1. Preheat oven to 350 degrees. Line a baking sheet with parchment paper and set aside.

2. Place dried cherries in a small bowl and cover with steaming-hot water for 10 minutes to rehydrate. Remove, pat dry, and set aside.

3. In a large mixing bowl, combine flours with baking powder and salt.

4. Cut butter into small cubes and cut into the flour mixture using a pastry cutter or two butter knives until mixture resembles coarse cornmeal. Toss cherries into dry mixture, making sure they are evenly distributed throughout the flour mixture.

5. In a separate bowl, whisk milk, egg, lemon zest, and agave until well combined. Fold the milk mixture into the flour mixture until well combined. Dough will be thick and slightly sticky. If necessary, use extra flour to gather the dough into a ball. Gently place on a floured surface and use your hands to pat the dough into a 1-inch-thick rectangle. Using a sharp knife, cut the dough horizontally once and then into thirds vertically, to make 6 squares. Cut each square again at an angle, to make 12 triangles.

Gently place each scone on prepared baking sheet. Brush the tops evenly with agave and almond flour.

6. Bake 20 to 22 minutes or until scones are firm and lightly browned on the bottom.

7. Serve warm or let cool completely and store in a cool, dry place overnight. (Scones can be frozen and reheated for up to a month. Reheat at 200 degrees for 10 minutes.)

▶ SERVES 12

tip: Keeping all ingredients—and your mixing bowls—cold creates a flaky texture in your scones.

featured ingredient

almond flour

To make almond flour, blanched almonds are ground into a fine meal. The flour is great to use in baked goods such as cookies, muffins, or dense cakes. Almond flour lends a sweet flavor, and adds protein and healthy fats. It also adds a soft, grainy texture, which makes cookies crispier and gives cakes or muffins a hearty, whole-grain feel. For best results, store almond flour in the freezer.

Pear-Rosemary Bread

NS

½ fresh pear

¾ cup spelt flour

½ cup oatmeal flour

1 tablespoon finely chopped fresh rosemary

½ teaspoon sea salt

2 teaspoons baking powder

2 large eggs

¼ cup agave

¼ cup extra virgin olive oil

⅓ cup chopped walnuts

1. Preheat oven to 350 degrees. Grease 8½" x 4½" loaf pan with oil from a refillable oil mister and set aside.

2. Peel and dice a ripe pear into small pieces and set out on a paper towel to drain excess water.

3. In a large bowl, whisk flours, rosemary, salt, and baking powder to combine.

4. In a separate bowl, whisk eggs, agave, and olive oil until well combined. Add the wet ingredients to the flour mixture and stir to combine. Fold in chopped walnuts and drained pears.

5. Spoon batter into prepared loaf pan. Bake 30 to 35 minutes, or until cake tester comes out clean.

▶ SERVES 10

tip: Refillable spray cans are widely available, so fill with allowable oil and use as nonstick spray.

Lunch

Each lunch recipe provides a balance between vegetables and varying types of proteins while staying lighter on the complex carbohydrates. Recipes that are more dominantly vegetable or protein include suggestions for a tasty complement of the other.

Navy Bean Hummus and Feta Sandwich **NS**

2 slices brown rice bread

½ teaspoon olive oil

Large-grain sea salt, to taste

2 tablespoons Navy Bean Hummus*

1 (¼-inch-thick) slice brick feta cheese

3 thin-sliced rounds green bell pepper

2 leaves Boston Bibb lettuce

1. Toast bread lightly until honey brown, and drizzle one side of each slice with olive oil and a scant sprinkling of sea salt.

2. Smear hummus on the olive oil side of one piece of toast, and top with feta, sliced bell peppers, and lettuce leaves. Place the second piece of toast oil side down, and slice in half.

3. Serve immediately.

*See Navy Bean Hummus **NS** (page 157).

▶ SERVES 2

1. Preheat oven to 400 degrees. Line a baking sheet with parchment paper and set aside.

2. Combine all meatball ingredients in a large bowl and gently combine with your hands. Try not to overwork the meat because it will get too tough.

3. Roll meatballs into golf ball–size pieces and place 2 inches apart on prepared baking sheet. Bake for 20 minutes or until golden brown and cooked through.

4. While meatballs cook, prepare pimiento sauce. In a high-sided skillet, heat olive oil over medium heat. Sauté onion and garlic, 5 to 6 minutes. Add chopped pimientos, agave, and stock and bring to a boil. Reduce to a gentle bubble, and let cook 10 to 15 minutes. Add salt, to taste.

5. When meatballs are done cooking, add to sauce and toss to coat. Spoon onto buns and top with cheese and basil.

6. Serve warm.

*See Basic Bread Crumbs **NS** recipe (page 211). See Vegetable Stock **NS** recipe (page 211).

▶ SERVES 4

meatballs:

1 pound lean, ground, organic lamb

¼ cup grated onion

⅓ cup finely chopped fresh mint

¼ teaspoon sea salt

1 teaspoon curry powder

1 large egg

5 tablespoons bread crumbs*

pimiento sauce:

2 teaspoons olive oil

½ cup onions, chopped

1 clove garlic, minced

1 (4.2-oz.) jar pimientos, drained and chopped

½ cup Vegetable Stock*

Sea salt, to taste

1 teaspoon agave

½ cup fresh basil, chopped

4 brown rice or millet buns

½ cup mozzarella

Fish Fillet Sandwich ^{NS}

fish:

- 1 pound haddock
- ¼ teaspoon sea salt
- 1 large egg, slightly beaten
- ½ cup spelt flour
- 1 teaspoon garlic powder
- 1 tablespoon olive oil

sauce:

- 1 (5.5-oz.) container thick low-fat Greek yogurt
- 1 tablespoon minced onion
- Sea salt, to taste
- 1 tablespoon chopped fresh dill
- 2 teaspoons lemon zest
- 4 spelt or brown rice buns
- 1 cup shredded romaine lettuce

1. Season haddock with sea salt, and slice into 4 individual fillets. In one large, flat-bottomed bowl, add beaten egg, and in a second combine flour and garlic powder. Dip each haddock fillet into the egg and then into the flour mixture. Dust off excess flour, and place onto a clean plate.

2. In a large, high-sided skillet, heat olive oil over medium heat. Add fish fillets, keeping 2 inches of space between each. Cook about 4 minutes per side or until center is flaky and opaque.

3. Make yogurt sauce by whisking all sauce ingredients in a small bowl.

4. Toast buns, spoon yogurt sauce on each bun half, and top with romaine and cooked fish.

▶ SERVES 4

tip: Keep an eye on the fish while it cooks to make sure it does not burn. You may need to flip the fish twice to make sure this does not happen. If more oil is needed, add 1 teaspoon at a time.

EAT RIGHT FOR YOUR TYPE PERSONALIZED COOKBOOK

2 teaspoons olive oil, divided

4 strips (nitrate- and preservative-free) turkey bacon

4 cups spinach

4 teaspoons ghee

4 slices oat bread

½ cup shredded mozzarella cheese

1. Preheat oven to 200 degrees.

2. Heat 1 teaspoon olive oil in a medium skillet over medium heat. Cook bacon for 1 to 2 minutes per side. Drain on paper towel and keep warm in oven until you are ready to add it to the grilled cheese. This will help the bacon crisp up further.

3. In same skillet, sauté spinach in remaining 1 teaspoon olive oil over medium heat for 1 to 2 minutes, just until leaves are wilted.

4. Spread ghee evenly on one side of each piece of bread. Place bacon, spinach, and cheese on unbuttered side of bread, and top with a second piece of buttered bread, so that the outer side of each piece is buttered. Cook in skillet over medium heat until lightly browned on each side and cheese has melted.

5. Slice in half and serve warm.

▶ SERVES 2

Greens and Beans Salad (NS)

salad:

1 head escarole

½ cup canned white beans, drained and rinsed

2 cups snap peas

4 cups string beans

dressing:

1 tablespoon fresh mint

1 tablespoon fresh lime juice

⅛ teaspoon ground cumin

1 clove garlic, minced

½ teaspoon honey

¼ cup olive oil

Sea salt, to taste

1. Wash escarole and pat dry. Tear escarole into bite-size pieces and place into a large serving bowl, top with white beans, and set aside.

2. Bring a large pot of water to boil. Boil snap peas and string beans for 3 minutes, drain, and shock in a large bowl of ice water to stop the cooking process. Lay the peas and beans on a kitchen towel to dry, and add to escarole mixture.

3. Whisk together all dressing ingredients in a small bowl. Drizzle over salad and serve.

▶ SERVES 4

1. Preheat oven to 375 degrees.

2. Spread goat cheese evenly on top of pizza crust, and bake 3 to 4 minutes until cheese begins to melt. Remove and let cool.

3. Increase oven temperature to 400 degrees. Cut broccoli into bite-size florets, place on a baking sheet, and toss with olive oil and sea salt. Bake for 20 minutes. Remove from oven and cool completely.

4. In a small bowl, whisk together all dressing ingredients. Drizzle over watercress, beets, broccoli, and almonds, and toss to combine.

5. Top crust with salad mixture and serve cold.

▶ SERVES 4

crust:

¼ cup shaved hard goat cheese

Store-bought spelt crust (with allowable grains)

salad:

1 head broccoli

1 teaspoon olive oil

Sea salt, to taste

2 cups watercress

1 cup beets, diced and roasted

1 tablespoon blanched, slivered almonds

dressing:

1 tablespoon fresh lemon juice

1 teaspoon minced onion

1 tablespoon olive oil

2 teaspoons diced fresh oregano

1. Preheat oven to 375 degrees.

2. Peel beet and parsnips. Dice beet into ½-inch cubes, and slice parsnips into ½-inch pieces. Remove outer leaves from cauliflower, and cut into bite-size florets. Toss vegetables with olive oil, and season with sea salt. Spread in a single layer on a baking sheet, and bake for 55 to 60 minutes, tossing halfway through. Vegetables should be easily pierced with fork and slightly browned on the edges and bottoms.

3. To prepare dressing, grate fresh horseradish. In a small bowl, whisk all dressing ingredients to combine.

4. Toss dandelion greens in a large bowl with horseradish dressing, top with roasted vegetables, and serve.

▶ SERVES 4

greens:

1 raw beet

2 parsnips

1 head cauliflower

2 teaspoons olive oil

2 bunches dandelion greens

Sea salt, to taste

dressing:

¼ cup olive oil

¼ cup grated fresh horseradish

1 tablespoon fresh, chopped basil

2 tablespoons fresh lemon juice

Sea salt, to taste

Roasted-Eggplant Greek Salad (NS)

salad:

2 cups cubed eggplant

2 teaspoons olive oil

Sea salt, to taste

6 cups torn romaine lettuce

½ cup sliced pepperoncini peppers

½ cup feta cheese, crumbled

dressing:

1 tablespoon fresh oregano

2 tablespoons fresh-squeezed lemon juice

3 tablespoons olive oil

Sea salt, to taste

1. Preheat oven to 375 degrees. Spray a baking sheet with non-stick cooking spray.

2. Place eggplant on prepared baking sheet. Drizzle with olive oil and sprinkle with sea salt. Bake for 35 minutes, until eggplant is softened and slightly browned on the bottom. Remove from oven, and let cool.

3. In the bottom of a large bowl, whisk dressing ingredients together, and set aside.

4. Wash lettuce, and pat dry. Tear into bite-size pieces, and place in a serving bowl. Add roasted eggplant, peppers, and feta cheese. Drizzle with dressing and toss to combine.

▶ SERVES 4

EAT RIGHT FOR YOUR TYPE PERSONALIZED COOKBOOK

1. Peel outer leaves of radicchio, and discard the first couple leaves. Continue peeling inner leaves gently, snapping at the base to maintain the integrity of each leaf. Clean with cold water and let dry on a kitchen towel.

2. Flake salmon into a bowl, and add chives, salt, peas, and apples.

3. In a small bowl, whisk together honey, oregano, lemon juice, lime zest, and olive oil. Drizzle over salmon mixture, and toss gently to combine.

4. Spoon salmon salad into prepared radicchio cups.

▶ SERVES 2

1 head radicchio

½ pound salmon, cooked

3 tablespoons chopped chives

½ teaspoon sea salt

½ cup cooked peas

½ cup finely diced apples

1 teaspoon honey

1 teaspoon chopped fresh oregano

Juice of 1 lemon

Zest of 1 lime

¼ cup olive oil

Baked Falafel NS

1½ cups dried navy beans (not canned or precooked)

1 tablespoon olive oil, divided

½ cup chopped parsley

2 tablespoons spelt flour

1 cup chopped onion

2 cloves garlic, minced

¼ teaspoon coriander

¼ teaspoon cumin

½ teaspoon sea salt

1. Soak dry beans overnight in cold water, drain, and rinse.

2. Boil presoaked beans for 30 minutes, drain, and rinse. Beans should be almost completely cooked, but remain a firm texture. Set beans in a single layer on a paper towel to dry.

3. Preheat oven to 350 degrees. Brush a baking sheet with 1 to 2 teaspoons olive oil, and set aside.

4. In a food processor, add beans, parsley, flour, onion, garlic, coriander, cumin, and salt. Pulse until ingredients form a thick paste. Use a tablespoon to scoop mixture into the palm of your hand and roll into balls and place on prepared baking sheet. Repeat until all of the mixture has been used. Brush remaining olive oil on the tops of falafel balls and bake for 25 minutes.

5. Increase the oven temperature to 400 degrees, and bake an additional 15 minutes. Falafels will be cooked through, warm and firm through the center.

6. Serve on top of Roasted-Eggplant Greek Salad.*

*See Roasted-Eggplant Greek Salad **NS** recipe (page 56).

▶ SERVES 4

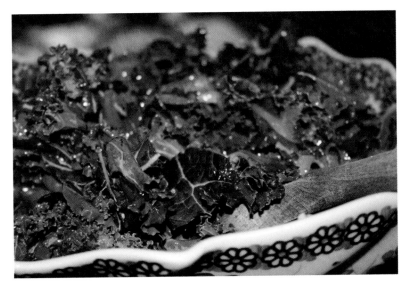

salad:

1 bunch kale

2 teaspoons olive oil

1 large white onion, sliced

½ cup raisins

dressing:

2 tablespoons olive oil

2 limes, juiced

1 clove garlic, minced

⅛ teaspoon ground cumin

Sea salt, to taste

1. Wash kale and dry on kitchen towels. Strip kale off the woody stems by holding the stem with one hand, wrapping finger and thumb of the other hand around the stem, and pulling quickly down. Discard stems and tear leaves into bite-size pieces. Place in a large bowl and set aside.

2. Heat olive oil in a skillet over medium heat. Add onion, and sauté 3 to 4 minutes. Add raisins, and continue cooking for 5 minutes. Remove from heat and toss with raw kale.

3. In a small bowl, whisk together dressing ingredients. Drizzle over kale salad and toss to coat. Serve with leftover or chilled baked salmon or beans for added protein.

▶ SERVES 4

Crunchy Vegetable Spring Rolls with Sweet Cherry Dip NS

spring rolls:

3 small, tricolored carrots

1 cup thinly sliced kale

1 orange bell pepper, thinly sliced

¼ cup finely sliced red onion

¼ cup julienned fresh basil

2 teaspoons olive oil

Sea salt, to taste

4 rice paper wraps

sweet cherry dip:

⅓ cup (no sugar added) cherry jam

1 tablespoon fresh grated ginger

1 tablespoon finely diced onion

1 teaspoon agave

Juice of ½ lemon

Sea salt, to taste

1. Peel and slice carrots into thin matchsticks.

2. Toss kale, bell pepper, carrots, onion, and basil together in a bowl with olive oil and sea salt, to taste. Set aside.

3. Pour hot water halfway up a large, flat-bottomed bowl. One at a time, submerge rice paper wraps in water until they soften and become pliable, about 30 seconds. Rice paper will be delicate, so be gentle. Place rice paper on a placemat or cutting board and spoon about 2 tablespoons vegetable mixture down the center of the rice paper. Roll the sides over the vegetables first and then pull the top over the vegetables and continue to roll up. Slice in half and repeat until remaining rice papers and filling are used.

4. In a small saucepan, combine all sauce ingredients over low heat. Stir 1 to 2 minutes until warmed through and melted together.

5. Serve wraps with cherry dip.

▶ SERVES 2

featured ingredient

rice paper wraps

Typically found in Asian markets, rice paper is used to make spring rolls, and thanks to its increased popularity, can now be found at most natural or health food stores. It is made of rice and water, and when dried, resembles stiffened parchment paper that looks pretty inedible. When soaked in warm water, however, rice paper transforms to a pliable, tender state, and can be used as a delicate wrap for fresh delicious flavors that get tucked inside like a burrito. Rice paper comes in packages of 50 to 100 papers and costs close to nothing, so it is a great, low-calorie, low-budget addition to your culinary repertoire.

Feta, Spinach, and Yellow Pepper Pie (NS)

crust:

2 tablespoons quinoa flour

⅓ cup millet flour

⅔ cup brown rice flour

½ teaspoon sea salt

4 tablespoons cold unsalted butter or ghee

5 tablespoons ice-cold water

filling:

2 teaspoons olive oil

4 cups baby spinach

2 cups chopped red kale

1 cup diced yellow pepper

½ cup diced white onion

1 cup feta cheese

2 large eggs

⅓ cup Vegetable Stock*

2 tablespoons fresh thyme

Sea salt, to taste

1. Preheat oven to 375 degrees.

2. Make crust by tossing flours and salt. Cut cold butter into small pieces and add to flour mixture. Using a crossing motion with two butter knives or a pastry cutter, incorporate butter into the flour until the mixture resembles coarse cornmeal. Add water, 1 tablespoon at a time, until the dough comes together but is not sticky. Gather dough in your hands and knead until it becomes smooth and pliable. Small pieces of butter should still be visible. Place in a bowl and cover dough with plastic wrap. Refrigerate 1 hour.

3. Roll dough on a flat, floured surface until about 12 inches in diameter and approximately ⅛-inch thick. Place into a 9-inch pie plate and gently press the dough into the pan, pinching edges between two fingers to create crimped edges.

4. Par-bake crust for 15 minutes. Par-baking means partially baking a crust to firm the crust before adding filling.

5. Prepare filling while crust bakes. Heat olive oil in large skillet over medium heat. Sauté spinach, kale, pepper, and onion for about 4 minutes, just until vegetables are tender. Transfer vegetables to a large bowl, toss with feta, and set aside to cool.

6. In a separate bowl, whisk eggs, stock, thyme, and sea salt, to taste. Pour over cooled vegetables, and mix to combine.

7. Pour filling into par-baked crust, and bake 30 minutes or until filling is firm.

8. Serve warm or cold (if serving cold, let cool and then place in refrigerator until ready to eat).

*See Vegetable Stock **NS** recipe (page 211).

▶ SERVES 6

Kidney Bean Stew

2 teaspoons olive oil

1 cup diced onion

1 celery root (celeriac), peeled and diced

2 cups diced orange bell pepper

2 cans organic kidney beans, drained and rinsed

1½ cups Vegetable Stock*

1 clove garlic

1 sprig sage

4 sprigs thyme

1 teaspoon sea salt

2 cups snow peas

1. In a large Dutch oven, heat olive oil over medium heat. Add onion and celery root, sautéing 4 to 5 minutes. Add orange pepper and sauté an additional 2 to 3 minutes. Vegetables should be tender and aromatic. Add remaining ingredients and bring to a gentle boil.

2. Reduce heat, cover, and simmer 25 minutes, until vegetables are soft and warmed through. Add snow peas and cook a final 5 minutes.

3. Remove sage and thyme sprigs, then serve warm.

*See Vegetable Stock **NS** recipe (page 211).

▶ SERVES 4

Dinner

The bulk of the recipes in this book are in this section. Here you will find a variety of dishes from pastas to seafood, all-in-one dishes, and so on. Most of the recipes are simple to make, but others take a bit more time to prepare. Hopefully these dishes inspire you to take some time to enjoy delicious, wholesome food for yourself and your family.

Mac and Cheese with Roasted Vegetables

1 large head broccoli

2 large red bell peppers

1 tablespoon olive oil

5 sprigs thyme, divided

Sea salt, to taste

1 tablespoon plus 2 teaspoons ghee, divided

½ cup bread crumbs*

2 tablespoons white or brown rice flour

2 cups Vegetable Stock*

1 cup 2 percent cow's milk

2 sprigs sage, chopped

1 pound brown rice or quinoa elbow pasta

1 cup shredded mozzarella cheese

½ cup cubed fresh mozzarella cheese

1. Preheat oven to 375 degrees.

2. Cut broccoli and bell peppers into bite-size pieces. Place in a single layer on a baking sheet, drizzle with olive oil, and salt. Strip leaves from thyme sprigs and sprinkle over the vegetables. Bake for 30 minutes, until the vegetables are tender and slightly browned. Set aside.

3. Melt 2 teaspoons ghee, toss with bread crumbs and a pinch of sea salt, and set aside.

4. Make a roux by melting remaining 1 tablespoon of ghee in a saucepan over medium-low heat and whisking in rice flour until well combined into a paste. Gradually add stock and milk to flour mixture, whisking after each addition until smooth and free of lumps. Add sage and increase heat to medium. Bring to a boil, whisking constantly. Reduce heat to a simmer and cook until the roux thickens, about 10 minutes. Add salt, to taste.

5. Cook pasta according to package instructions (if using brown rice pasta, cook 3 to 4 minutes short of recommended cooking time). Drain pasta and pour into casserole dish. Toss with roasted vegetables. Cover pasta with sauce and shredded mozzarella cheese, gently tossing with pasta to incorporate throughout the dish. Top with reserved bread crumbs and fresh mozzarella.

6. Bake 20 to 25 minutes, until hot and bubbling, and the bread crumbs are golden brown and toasted.

*See Basic Bread Crumbs **NS** recipe (page 211). See Vegetable Stock **NS** recipe (page 211).

▶ SERVES 6

EAT RIGHT FOR YOUR TYPE PERSONALIZED COOKBOOK

1. Bring a large pot of salted water to a boil. Cook spaghetti according to package directions (if using brown rice spaghetti, cook 4 minutes short of package cooking time). Drain, reserving ½ cup pasta cooking water, and set aside.

2. Heat olive oil in a large, high-sided skillet over medium heat. Sauté onions for 4 to 5 minutes. Chop turkey bacon into about ¼-inch pieces and add to the pan, sautéing until browned, about 5 to 6 minutes. Remove turkey bacon and onions and set aside.

3. Slice asparagus spears in quarters and add to skillet with kale. Sauté until vegetables are tender, about 3 to 4 minutes. Add bacon and onion back to the skillet and reduce heat to low.

4. In a bowl, whisk together eggs, yolks, milk, and salt, to taste. Slowly pour reserved pasta cooking water into the egg mixture to temper the eggs. Remove the skillet from the heat, add cooked pasta to vegetables, and pour egg mixture over top. The heat from the pasta will gently cook the eggs and create a sauce. Stir in cheese and season with salt.

5. Serve immediately.

▶ SERVES 6

1 pound spelt or brown rice spaghetti

2 teaspoons olive oil

½ cup diced onions

4 slices turkey bacon

2 cups asparagus

3 cups sliced red kale

2 large eggs

2 egg yolks

¼ cup 2 percent cow's milk

Sea salt, to taste

¼ cup ricotta cheese

1. Preheat oven to 375 degrees.

2. Tear beet greens into bite-size pieces and place them in a large bowl. Snap asparagus spears close to the bottom, and discard the woody stems. Cut into bite-size pieces and toss with beet greens. Tear 1½ bunches kale into large bite-size pieces and add to bowl. Toss vegetables with 2 teaspoons olive oil and a pinch of salt.

3. Place on a baking sheet, and bake for 12 minutes or until vegetables are tender and kale has slightly crispy edges. Set aside. Reduce oven temperature to 200 degrees.

4. Bring a large pot of water to boil. Cook pasta 4 minutes short of recommended cooking time.

5. While pasta is cooking, prepare pesto. Tear remaining kale into bite-size pieces; you'll have about 2½ cups. Combine with ½ cup olive oil, lemon juice, walnuts, garlic, salt, and pepper in a food processor, and pulse until smooth. Spoon into a bowl and set aside.

6. Cook bacon in a skillet with remaining 1 teaspoon olive oil until crispy, about 2 minutes per side. Wrap in a damp paper towel and keep warm in the oven until ready to serve, to make bacon extra crispy.

7. Drain pasta and place in a large pasta bowl. Toss immediately with pesto, cheese, peas, and roasted vegetables. Sprinkle with cracked red pepper and lemon zest. Crumble bacon and sprinkle on top. Serve warm.

▶ SERVES 6

1 bunch asparagus

1 bunch beet greens

2 large bunches kale, divided

½ cup plus 3 teaspoons olive oil

Sea salt, to taste

1 pound brown rice pasta

Juice of 1 lemon

½ cup walnuts

2 cloves garlic, minced

½ teaspoon cracked red pepper, plus extra for serving

3 slices nitrate- / preservative-free turkey bacon

½ cup Gouda cheese, grated

2 cups cooked peas

Zest of 1 lemon

Sweet Potato Gnocchi with Basil-Cranberry Sauce (NS)

gnocchi:

2 cups sweet potato, boiled

¾ cup brown rice flour

¼ cup millet flour

1 teaspoon sea salt

1 large egg, beaten

¼ teaspoon fresh ground nutmeg

sauce:

1 tablespoon olive oil

1 teaspoon ghee

¼ cup finely diced shallots

½ cup Vegetable Stock*

1 tablespoon lemon juice

¼ cup dried cranberries

½ cup torn fresh basil

1. Mash boiled sweet potatoes with a fork or potato masher until smooth and creamy.

2. In a large bowl, combine smashed sweet potatoes with remaining gnocchi ingredients. Use your hands to lightly form into a dough ball. If the dough is too sticky, sprinkle more brown rice flour over the dough. Grab a handful of dough at a time and roll on a floured surface into long, ¾-inch-thick cylinders. Repeat with remaining dough.

3. Use a sharp knife to slice the cylinders into 1-inch pieces. Roll each piece gently over the back of a fork, to make indentations in the gnocchi.

4. Bring a large pot of salted water to a gentle boil. Drop gnocchi into the water in batches, being careful to not crowd the pot. The gnocchi will float to the top when they are finished cooking, about 2 to 3 minutes. Remove with a slotted spoon and transfer to a baking sheet until all gnocchi has been cooked.

5. Heat olive oil and ghee in a large skillet over medium heat. Sauté shallots for 2 to 3 minutes. Add stock, lemon juice, and cranberries.

6. Toss gnocchi with sauce just to coat, garnish with basil, and serve warm.

*See Vegetable Stock **NS** recipe (page 211).

▶ SERVES 4

EAT RIGHT FOR YOUR TYPE PERSONALIZED COOKBOOK

1. In a small skillet, combine all infused oil ingredients. Cook over low heat for 15 minutes. Remove from heat and set aside.

2. In a food processor or mini chopper, combine ¼ cup almonds, olive oil, sage, cheese, spinach, lemon juice, lemon zest, sea salt, and water. Pulse until mixture is pureed and resembles a thick sauce.

3. Cook pasta according to package instructions. If using brown rice pasta, cook 4 minutes short of package instructions.

4. While the pasta cooks, heat grill pan over medium heat and brush with infused oil. Peel outer layers of radicchio and discard. Cut peeled radicchio in quarters. Brush each quarter with infused olive oil, and grill about 1 minute per side or until radicchio begins to become tender and slightly wilted.

5. Drain pasta, and toss with pesto and kefir in a large serving bowl. Top with grilled radicchio and reserved toasted almonds.

6. Serve immediately.

▶ SERVES 2

tip: Store infused oil in a sealed, glass container in a cool, dry place for up to 1 week. Great on salads or drizzled over toast.

infused oil:

Zest of ½ lemon

⅓ cup olive oil

⅛ teaspoon mustard powder

½ teaspoon cumin seeds

2 cloves garlic, smashed

pesto:

¼ cup plus 2 tablespoons toasted almonds, divided

2 tablespoons olive oil

¼ cup chopped fresh sage

¼ cup grated hard goat cheese

1 cup chopped spinach

2 tablespoons lemon juice

1 teaspoon lemon zest

½ teaspoon sea salt

1 tablespoon water

¾ pound spinach, brown-rice, or spelt spaghetti

2 heads radicchio

½ cup kefir cheese, cut into 1-inch dice

1. Preheat oven to 375 degrees.

2. Trim ends off zucchini and slice in 4 long pieces, about ¼-inch thick.

3. Line zucchini and portabella mushrooms in a single layer on baking sheets. Drizzle evenly with 2 tablespoons olive oil and 1 teaspoon sea salt. Roast on top rack of oven for 20 minutes.

4. Heat remaining 2 teaspoons oil in a large skillet over medium heat. Sauté onion for 8 to 10 minutes, until tender and translucent. Add spinach and sauté 1 minute, just until spinach wilts. Remove from heat.

5. In a large bowl, stir together ricotta cheese, walnuts, egg, cloves, and reserved spinach mixture. Set aside.

6. Remove vegetables from the oven, and let cool while you make the pesto. Reduce oven temperature to 350 degrees.

7. Place all pesto ingredients in a blender and pulse until smooth.

8. Assemble lasagna by layering a thin layer of pesto in the bottom of a 9" x 11" baking dish, topped with a layer of roasted zucchini, a layer of ricotta mixture, ½ cup mozzarella cheese, pesto, mushrooms, ricotta, pesto, remaining zucchini, remaining ricotta, remaining pesto, and remaining mozzarella cheese.

9. Bake for 25 minutes until cheese is melted and slightly browned on the top. Serve warm.

▶ SERVES 6

lasagna:

5 medium zucchini

6 portabella mushrooms

2 tablespoons plus 2 teaspoons olive oil

1½ teaspoons sea salt, divided

1 cup finely diced onion

4 cups packed baby spinach

2 cups part-skim ricotta cheese

½ cup finely chopped walnuts

1 large egg

Dash of cloves

1 cup shredded mozzarella cheese

pesto:

2 cups packed baby spinach

2 cups packed basil

½ teaspoon sea salt

2 cloves garlic

¼ cup lemon juice

¼ cup olive oil

¼ cup walnuts

2 tablespoons water

Noodles with Poached Salmon and Creamy Basil Sauce NS

2 cups Vegetable Stock*
2 cups water
1 lemon, sliced
1½ pounds salmon
1 pound spelt pasta
Spicy mustard, for serving (optional)

sauce:

2 cups spinach
1 cup basil
1 clove garlic, minced
1 cup northern beans
2 teaspoons lemon zest
½ cup Vegetable Stock*
1 teaspoon granulated mustard

1. Fill a high-sided skillet with stock, water, and lemon slices. Bring to a simmer and add salmon. Cover and cook 12 to 15 minutes.

2. In the meantime, cook pasta according to package instructions.

3. While pasta and salmon cook, make sauce by pureeing sauce ingredients in a food processor or blender.

4. Drain pasta and toss with all but ¼ cup of the basil sauce. Top with salmon and drizzle with remaining sauce and spicy mustard, if desired.

5. Serve immediately.

*See Vegetable Stock NS recipe (page 211).

▶ SERVES 4

1 pound wild-caught salmon fillets

2 teaspoons olive oil, divided

½ teaspoon sea salt

Zest of 1 lemon

1 tablespoon lemon juice

2 tablespoons fresh grated ginger

1 teaspoon honey

1. Preheat oven to 400 degrees.

2. Rub salmon with 1 teaspoon olive oil and season with sea salt.

3. In a small bowl, mix lemon zest, lemon juice, remaining 1 teaspoon olive oil, ginger, and honey until combined. Brush evenly over the top of salmon.

4. Bake for 10 to 12 minutes.

5. Serve with Grilled Garlic-Ginger Bok Choy NS (page 127).

▶ SERVES 2

Salmon and Bean Cakes with Cilantro-Cream Sauce NS

1 pound cooked wild-caught salmon

1 cup cooked cannellini beans, drained and rinsed

1 teaspoon chopped scallions

1 teaspoon fresh rosemary

1 teaspoon fresh thyme

Sea salt, to taste

1 large egg, slightly beaten

½ cup bread crumbs*

2 teaspoons olive oil

sauce:

2 tablespoons walnuts

2 tablespoons olive oil

2 tablespoons hot water

¼ cup cilantro

Sea salt and pepper, to taste

1. Flake cooked salmon into a bowl, and carefully remove any bones. Add beans, scallions, rosemary, thyme, and sea salt. Gently stir in egg and bread crumbs.

2. Heat olive oil in skillet over medium heat. Form salmon mixture into patties, until all the mixture is used. Cook 3 to 4 minutes, flip, and cook an additional 3 to 4 minutes on the opposite side.

3. In a food processor, pulse walnuts until they form a paste. With the processor running, add olive oil and water. Once creamy, add cilantro, salt, and pepper.

4. Serve salmon cakes warm, drizzled with cilantro-cream sauce.

*See Basic Bread Crumbs NS recipe (page 211).

▶ SERVES 4

Baked Mahimahi with Crunchy Fennel Salad NS

1. Preheat oven to 350 degrees.

2. Season mahimahi with coriander, lemon zest, and ¼ teaspoon sea salt. Bake for 12 to 15 minutes or until fish is flaky and white.

3. While the seafood bakes, whisk parsley, olive oil, sea salt, to taste, lemon zest, and juice in the bottom of a bowl. Add fennel and apple, and toss to combine.

4. Plate fish, top with fennel salad, and serve immediately.

▶ SERVES 2

1 pound mahimahi

⅛ teaspoon ground coriander

1 teaspoon lemon zest

¼ teaspoon sea salt

fennel salad:

2 teaspoons chopped fresh parsley

2 teaspoons olive oil

Sea salt, to taste

1 teaspoon lemon zest

2 teaspoons lemon juice

2 cups thinly sliced fennel

1 cup thinly sliced Granny Smith apples

Parchment-Baked Snapper (NS)

1 pound snapper
(4 fillets)

½ teaspoon sea salt

½ teaspoon chili powder

2 cloves garlic, minced

1 tablespoon olive oil

1 cup thinly sliced peaches

1 cup thinly sliced red onion

½ cup sliced orange bell peppers

1. Preheat oven to 350 degrees.

2. Cut 4 12-inch x 12-inch pieces of parchment paper. Place snapper in the center of each piece of parchment paper, season with salt, chili powder, garlic, and olive oil. Top with peaches, onions, and bell peppers.

3. Lift side of parchment paper up, fold the edges together, and crease. Starting at the edges, crimp and pinch parchment to seal around the fish.

4. Bake 15 minutes or until fish is flaky and opaque. Serve warm.

▶ SERVES 4

EAT RIGHT FOR YOUR TYPE PERSONALIZED COOKBOOK

1 pound wild-caught halibut steak

1 teaspoon olive oil

½ teaspoon sea salt

¼ cup fig jam

2 tablespoons chopped fresh basil

2 teaspoons lemon zest

1 teaspoon lemon juice

1. Preheat oven to 400 degrees.

2. Slice halibut into 2 fillets. Drizzle with olive oil and sea salt.

3. In a small bowl, whisk together remaining ingredients. Spread evenly over top of halibut and place in a baking dish.

4. Bake for 30 minutes or until center is flaky and opaque.

▶ SERVES 2

Spicy Seafood Stew NS

1–2 dried ancho chili peppers

¼ cup wakame (optional)

2 teaspoons olive oil

1 cup diced onions

1 bulb fennel, diced

1 red bell pepper, diced

1 jalapeno, finely diced

½ teaspoon turmeric

½ teaspoon fennel seeds

Sea salt, to taste

2 (6½-oz.) cans pimiento

2 bay leaves

2 cups Vegetable Stock*

2 cups water

¾ pound cod

½ pound wild-caught salmon

1. Place dried ancho chilies in hot water for 10 to 12 minutes. If using wakame, place in cold water for 10 minutes.

2. In a stockpot, heat olive oil over medium heat. Sauté onion and fennel in olive oil for 4 to 5 minutes. Add red bell pepper and jalapeno, and sauté an additional 3 to 4 minutes. Season with turmeric, fennel seeds, and sea salt, to taste.

3. Drain chilies, discard stems and seeds, and set aside.

4. Drain and rinse wakame, if using, and immediately add to stockpot.

5. Drain pimientos and pat dry. Puree in a food processor with rehydrated chilies until very smooth. (Use less ancho chilies if you wish to reduce the spice.) Add pimiento mixture and bay leaves to sautéed vegetables with stock and water. Simmer 30 minutes.

6. While the stew simmers, dice cod and salmon into bite-size pieces. After the stew cooks for 30 minutes, add the seafood and let cook an additional 10 minutes, or until seafood is cooked through.

7. Serve warm.

*See Vegetable Stock NS recipe (page 211).

▶ SERVES 4

 Type B

featured ingredient

wakame

If you've had miso soup, you've most likely eaten wakame. Wakame is a nutrient-rich seaweed cultivated off the coast of Japan, and adds a briny finish to soups, stews, and even salads. It is most often dehydrated for distribution, but once soaked, returns to its dark-green color and velvety texture. Due to its mild flavor, wakame is a perfect way to begin adding seaweed to your diet. (In the picture, the wakame is in its dehydrated form.)

Seafood Paella

NS

3 teaspoons olive oil, divided

2 cups chopped yellow onion

1 cup diced carrots

2 cups diced red bell pepper

1 jalapeno, diced

2 teaspoons garlic, minced

1½ cups long-grain brown rice

15 threads saffron

1 teaspoon sea salt, plus more, to taste

1 teaspoon paprika

⅛ teaspoon cayenne pepper

¼ cup chopped parsley

2 cups Vegetable Stock*

1 cup water

1 bay leaf

2 teaspoons fresh oregano

¾ pound halibut fillets

¾ pound mahimahi fillets

1 teaspoon dried oregano

1. Preheat oven to 350 degrees.

2. In a large Dutch oven or paella pan, heat 1 teaspoon olive oil over medium heat. Sauté onion, carrots, bell peppers, jalapeno, and garlic for 6 to 7 minutes, stirring frequently. Vegetables should become tender, but not brown. Remove vegetables from pan and set aside.

3. Add remaining olive oil to the same pan, and toast rice for 2 minutes, stirring constantly. After 2 minutes, the rice will start to smell slightly nutty and darken in color. Add saffron, sea salt, paprika, and cayenne pepper.

4. Return vegetables to the Dutch oven with the rice and stir to combine. Add parsley, stock, water, bay leaf, and oregano. Bring to a simmer and cover. Place in preheated oven for 40 minutes.

5. While the paella cooks, dice seafood into 1-inch pieces, and toss with dried oregano and sea salt, to taste.

6. After 40 minutes, remove paella from oven, and add seafood pieces. Re-cover and bake an additional 12 minutes, until rice absorbs all the liquid.

7. Seafood should be flaky and opaque when fully cooked, and rice will be fluffy and tender.

8. Serve warm.

*See Vegetable Stock **NS** recipe (page 211).

▶ SERVES 6

1. Preheat oven to 350 degrees. Drizzle a 9" x 11" baking dish with olive oil to create a nonstick surface for the halibut, and set aside.

2. In a mini chopper or food processor, puree garlic with parsley, lemon zest, sea salt, and 2 teaspoons olive oil. Set aside.

3. Season halibut with sea salt. In a large skillet, heat 1 teaspoon olive oil over medium-high heat. Sear halibut, flesh side down for 2 minutes, just to create a crispy crust on the fish. Remove, place skin-side down in prepared baking dish, and top with parsley puree. Set aside.

4. To the same skillet, add onions, carrots, and cabbage. Sauté over medium heat in the remaining olive oil for about 5 minutes to soften the vegetables slightly. Add salt, to taste. Add stock and stir to deglaze bottom of pan. Pour the carrot mixture around the halibut in the baking dish. Cover and bake 12 minutes (cooking time will vary based on the thickness of the fish). Remove cover and continue to bake for an additional 5 minutes. Halibut should be flaky and bright white all the way through.

5. Remove dish from the oven. If sauce is runny, remove fish and vegetables and set aside, place the baking dish over medium heat on the stovetop, and stir the liquid to thicken the sauce.

6. Serve warm.

*See Vegetable Stock **NS** recipe (page 211).

▶ SERVES 4

4 teaspoons olive oil, divided, plus more for greasing

2 cloves garlic

¼ cup parsley

1 teaspoon lemon zest

1 teaspoon sea salt

1½ pounds halibut, skin on

1 red onion

2 white onions, chopped

3 large carrots, peeled and chopped

2 cups green cabbage, shredded

¼ cup fish stock or Vegetable Stock*

1. In a small bowl, combine chili powder, cumin, salt, paprika, and 1 tablespoon olive oil. Slice fish into 1-inch cubes, place in a large bowl, and drizzle spice mixture over fish. Marinate in the refrigerator for at least 20 minutes.

2. While the fish marinates, make the mango salad. Peel rind and pith off the lime. Carefully cut lime sections away from membrane with a paring knife. Place lime sections and all remaining salad ingredients in a large bowl, toss to combine, and set aside. Allowing the salad to sit while preparing the rest of the dish enables the flavors to combine and textures to soften slightly.

3. To prepare taco crêpes, whisk all crêpe ingredients together in a large bowl. Heat a large skillet or crêpe pan over medium to medium-high heat. (If not using a nonstick pan, use a nonstick cooking spray.) Once hot, spoon ¼ cup of the crêpe batter onto the skillet and quickly turn the skillet to spread batter in a very thin layer. Let cook about 1 minute, or until the edges start to pull away from the skillet and tiny bubbles appear in the center of the crêpe. Using a large, flat spatula or carefully lifting edges with your hands, flip the crêpe, and cook 1 additional minute on the other side. Repeat with remaining batter. Stack crêpe on a plate and keep warm until serving.

4. Brush a heated grill pan with remaining 1 teaspoon olive oil, and grill fish 2 to 3 minutes per side, until fish is flaky and opaque.

5. To assemble tacos, place taco crêpe on a plate and top with fish and mango salad.

6. Serve immediately.

▶ SERVES 4

fish:

¼ teaspoon chili powder

⅛ teaspoon cumin

½ teaspoon salt

¼ teaspoon paprika

1 tablespoon plus 1 teaspoon olive oil, divided

1 pound mahimahi

mango salad:

1 finely sliced fennel bulb

1 tablespoon chopped fresh mint

½ teaspoon lime zest

1 lime

2 teaspoons olive oil

½ cup diced mango

½ cup cooked northern beans, drained and rinsed

¼ teaspoon sea salt

taco crêpes:

2 eggs

½ teaspoon sea salt

⅔ cup brown rice flour

⅓ cup spelt flour

1 tablespoon olive oil

1½ cups 2 percent cow's milk

1. Preheat oven to 350 degrees.

2. Finely chop fresh herbs and place in a small bowl. Set aside.

3. Heat butter and 2 teaspoons olive oil in a large skillet over medium heat. Sauté shallots for 2 to 3 minutes. Add figs and kale, and sauté an additional 4 to 5 minutes. Remove from heat, mix in Parmesan cheese, and set aside.

4. Slice turkey breast in half to create two pieces. Butterfly turkey breasts by placing on a cutting board and carefully slicing horizontally through the meat, leaving a 1-inch border. This opens the breast so that stuffing it is made simple. Divide kale stuffing evenly between turkey breasts. Gently pull turkey back together and fasten with toothpicks. Sprinkle both sides of stuffed turkey breasts with reserved herb mixture.

5. Heat oven-safe skillet over medium heat, and add remaining olive oil. Sear stuffed turkey breasts, 3 to 4 minutes per side. Transfer skillet to oven and bake for 8 to 10 minutes or until juices run clear and the internal temperature of the turkey reaches 165 degrees.

6. Remove turkey from pan and set on a cutting board to rest. Place baking dish over medium heat and add flour and remaining 1 tablespoon butter, whisking into a paste. Slowly add stock, whisking constantly to form a gravy. Bring to a simmer and cook 2 to 3 minutes, until the gravy coats the back of a spoon.

7. Slice turkey breasts and drizzle with gravy. Serve warm.

*See Turkey Stock **NS** recipe (page 210).

▶ SERVES 4

1 tablespoon fresh oregano

2 tablespoons fresh thyme

2 tablespoons fresh basil

1 tablespoon plus 1 teaspoon butter, divided

1 tablespoon olive oil, divided

½ cup shallots, minced

¾ cup chopped figs

2 cups chopped kale

¼ cup Parmesan cheese (**NS** omit Parmesan cheese)

1 large, boneless turkey breast

1 tablespoon brown rice flour

1 cup Turkey* or Vegetable Stock*

Broccolini-Stuffed Turkey (NS)

2 teaspoons ghee

1 bunch broccolini, roughly chopped

½ red onion, diced

Sea salt, to taste

¼ cup walnuts

⅓ cup feta cheese, crumbled

1 cup Vegetable Stock*, divided

1 pound turkey tenderloin

1 tablespoon olive oil

1 tablespoon brown rice flour

1 tablespoon oregano

1 tablespoon lemon juice

1. Preheat oven to 350 degrees.

2. Heat ghee in a large skillet over medium heat. Sauté broccolini and onion until slightly tender, about 2 to 3 minutes. Season with salt, to taste.

3. Transfer broccolini mixture to a food processor. Add walnuts, cheese, and ¼ cup Vegetable Stock, and pulse to combine. Filling should be thick and pasty but not too dry, similar in consistency to cookie dough. If mixture looks dry, add additional stock, 1 tablespoon at a time.

4. Butterfly the turkey tenderloin by positioning the tenderloin with the tip facing you and the thickest part of the meat facing your slicing hand. Put your hand on top of the tenderloin and insert the knife into the thickest part of the meat, carefully cutting across the tenderloin almost until you reach the opposite side. This will create a pocket for the filling.

5. Spoon broccolini stuffing into tenderloin and secure closed with toothpicks or cooking twine. Season tenderloin with salt.

6. Heat olive oil in an oven-safe skillet over medium-high heat. Sear tenderloin, about 2 minutes per side. Cover and place in oven for 20 to 25 minutes. Turkey is cooked when juices run clear and the internal temperature reaches 165 degrees.

7. Remove turkey from skillet and set aside to rest. Return skillet to stovetop and place over medium heat. Add flour and gradually whisk in remaining stock, oregano, and lemon juice. Bring to a bubble and cook until thickened, about 5 minutes. Season gravy with sea salt if needed, and serve over turkey.

*See Vegetable Stock **NS** recipe (page 211).

▶ SERVES 4

EAT RIGHT FOR YOUR TYPE PERSONALIZED COOKBOOK

broccolini

Broccolini looks like an elongated and tender version of broccoli. Broccolini has a slightly milder taste, however, and is much more palatable when sautéed, roasted, or grilled. If cooked simply, it pairs best with olive oil and garlic. It is often confused with rappini or broccoli rabe, which has a much more bitter taste and is less appealing to some people.

1. Grind rice cakes in a food processor or mini chopper until they are small crumbs. Pour in a shallow bowl and add cheese, paprika, and salt. Toss to combine.

2. In another shallow bowl, whisk together egg and milk. Dip tenderloins in egg mixture and then into rice cake mixture, turning to coat each side.

3. Preheat oven to 375 degrees. Grease a baking sheet with non-stick cooking spray and set aside.

4. Heat oil in a large, oven-safe skillet over medium heat. Brown tenderloins, about 5 minutes per side. Place onto prepared baking sheet, and bake until cooked through, about 8 minutes or until the internal temperature reaches 165 degrees.

5. While the turkey cooks, make the dipping sauce by whisking together mustard, apricot spread, and lemon juice.

6. Serve warm.

▶ SERVES 4

tip: If you do not have an oven-safe skillet, simply wrap plastic handle with tinfoil.

tenders:

2 rice cakes

2 tablespoons Parmesan cheese (NS omit Parmesan cheese)

1 teaspoon sweet paprika

½ teaspoon sea salt

1 egg

2 teaspoons 2 percent cow's milk

4 turkey tenderloins

1 tablespoon olive oil

dipping sauce:

2 teaspoons dry mustard

2 tablespoons (no sugar added) apricot spread

1 teaspoon lemon juice

Shredded Turkey Bake

3 teaspoons olive oil, divided

1 cup diced carrots

1 cup diced onion

1 cup diced red bell pepper

2 tablespoons plus 1 teaspoon fresh thyme

2 cups carrot juice

1 cup Vegetable Stock*

⅛ teaspoon salt, plus additional, to taste

1½ pounds turkey tenderloin

1 tablespoon arrowroot starch

2 tablespoons cold water

½ cup quinoa

1 cup bread crumbs*

¼ cup shredded mozzarella cheese

¼ cup Parmesan cheese (NS omit Parmesan cheese or substitute more shredded mozzarella cheese)

1. Heat 2 teaspoons olive oil in a Dutch oven over medium heat. Add carrots and onion, and sauté for 5 minutes. Add 2 tablespoons thyme, carrot juice, stock, and salt. Stir just to combine and add turkey tenderloin. Bring to a boil, reduce heat to a low simmer, cover, and cook for 1½ hours.

2. Preheat oven to 375 degrees.

3. After 1½ hours, remove turkey, place onto a cutting board, and shred into bite-size pieces. Return to the pot and increase heat to medium, letting the carrot juice reduce slightly. In a small bowl, dissolve arrowroot starch in water. Add to shredded turkey mixture and stir to help the liquid thicken. After 10 minutes, add quinoa and cook an additional 12 minutes.

4. Mix bread crumbs with 1 teaspoon olive oil, ⅛ teaspoon salt, and remaining 1 teaspoon fresh thyme. Toss with cheese.

5. Spoon turkey mixture into 6 individual (7-oz.) ramekins, top with bread crumbs and cheese mixture, and bake for 8 to 10 minutes or until turkey mixture is bubbling and topping is melted.

*See Vegetable Stock **NS** recipe (page 211). See Basic Bread Crumbs **NS** recipe (page 211).

▶ SERVES 6

Green Tea–Poached Turkey Tenderloins NS

1. In a high-sided skillet, bring 4 cups water to a boil, and steep the tea bags for 3 minutes. Reduce heat to medium, and add turkey. Slice half the lemon and add to the poaching liquid with sea salt. Cover and let cook 18 to 20 minutes or until internal temperature of turkey reaches 165 degrees.

2. Puree parsley, olive oil, garlic, juice from the remaining half of the lemon, and water in a food processor until very smooth.

3. Serve turkey warm, topped with parsley oil.

▶ SERVES 4

8 green tea bags

1 pound turkey tenderloins

1 lemon, divided

½ teaspoon sea salt

1 cup fresh parsley

3 tablespoons olive oil

1 clove garlic

1 tablespoon water

Turkey Pot Pie with Crunchy Topping NS

filling:

2 teaspoons olive oil

1 cup frozen pearl onions, thawed

1 cup diced baby carrots

1 cup frozen sweet peas, thawed

1 cup diced parsnips

2 tablespoons spelt or oat flour

3¼ cups Turkey Stock* or Vegetable Stock*

1½ pounds roasted turkey breast, shredded

¼ teaspoon saffron threads

½ teaspoon dry mustard

topping:

1 teaspoon olive oil

2 cups bread crumbs*

2 teaspoons ghee, melted

Sea salt, to taste

crust:

Spelt or whole-wheat store-bought crust (containing allowable grains)

1. Preheat oven to 375 degrees.

2. In a Dutch oven, heat 2 teaspoons olive oil over medium heat. Sauté onions, carrots, peas, and parsnips for 5 minutes until vegetables just begin to soften. Sprinkle flour over vegetables and add stock, stirring to prevent lumps. Add roasted turkey, saffron, and dry mustard, stirring to combine. Cover and let cook 15 minutes, stirring occasionally.

3. In the meantime, sauté bread crumbs in 1 teaspoon olive oil and ghee for 3 to 4 minutes. Remove and toss bread crumbs with sea salt, to taste.

4. Uncover turkey filling, spoon into spelt crust, and top with toasted bread crumbs. Place in the oven for 20 minutes. The crust will be browned around the edges and the turkey mixture should be hot and bubbling.

5. Serve warm.

tip: I use leftover roasted turkey for this recipe, but if you're roasting from scratch, place a bone-in, skin-on turkey breast on a rack in a roasting pan. Top with your favorite fresh, chopped herbs and bake for 1½ to 2 hours, until the internal temperature reaches 165 degrees.

*See Turkey Stock **NS** recipe (page 210). See Basic Bread Crumbs **NS** recipe (page 211).

▶ SERVES 8

EAT RIGHT FOR YOUR TYPE PERSONALIZED COOKBOOK

2 teaspoons olive oil

1 pound turkey breast

2 cups diced onion

2 cups diced parsnips

2 large sprigs fresh rosemary

4 large sprigs fresh thyme

1 cup water

1 cup Vegetable Stock*

4 cups torn red kale

1. Preheat slow cooker to medium.

2. Heat olive oil in a large skillet over medium heat, and sear turkey breast on all sides. Remove from heat and set aside.

3. In the same skillet, add onion and parsnips, and sauté 3 to 4 minutes. Remove from skillet and place in bottom of slow cooker with rosemary and thyme. Place turkey breast on top of vegetables and herbs.

4. Add water and stock to skillet used to sear turkey and increase heat to medium-high to deglaze, scraping up all the bits. Pour liquid and bits over turkey in the slow cooker.

5. Cover and cook 1 hour. Add the kale and cook 1 additional hour.

6. Serve warm.

*See Vegetable Stock **NS** recipe (page 211).

▶ SERVES 4

1. Preheat oven to 325 degrees.

2. In a large skillet over medium heat, heat ghee. Sauté garlic and onion for 4 to 5 minutes, until tender and slightly browned. Add cumin, sea salt, and chili powder, stir, and cook an additional 2 minutes. Add pimiento puree, stock, and almond butter, stir to combine, and cook 3 to 4 minutes.

3. Remove from heat, stir in chocolate, and transfer mixture to a food processor. Puree until smooth. As an optional step, push mole sauce through a strainer to have a silky smooth sauce. If you do not mind the texture, however, leave it as is.

4. Set aside ⅓ of the sauce for use after cooking. Remove skin from turkey drumsticks, discard, and coat drumsticks with mole sauce. Place in a baking dish, cover, and bake for 1 to 1½ hours. Check internal temperature to make sure it reaches 165 degrees.

5. Once cooked, remove from oven and serve warm, topped with reserved mole sauce.

*See Vegetable Stock **NS** recipe (page 211).

▶ SERVES 2

1 teaspoon ghee

2 cloves garlic, minced

¼ cup diced onion

1 teaspoon ground cumin

1 teaspoon sea salt

2 teaspoons ancho chili powder

¼ cup pureed pimiento peppers

¼ cup Vegetable Stock*

2 teaspoons almond butter

1 ounce 100 percent dark chocolate, shaved

3 turkey drumsticks

Turkey-Ginger Stir-Fry (NS)

3 teaspoons olive oil, divided

1 (2-inch) piece ginger, peeled and thinly sliced

¾ pound turkey breast, thinly sliced

2 cups snow peas

1 cup sliced bok choy

¼ cup finely sliced orange bell pepper

⅓ cup plum jam

1 tablespoon lemon juice

1 tablespoon lemon zest

1 tablespoon agave

1. In a large wok or sauté pan, heat 2 teaspoons olive oil over medium heat. Add ginger and sauté 1 minute. Add turkey and stir-fry until cooked, about 3 to 4 minutes. Remove from wok and set aside.

2. Add remaining olive oil, snow peas, bok choy, and peppers. Stir-fry 3 to 4 minutes. Add turkey back to the wok along with remaining ingredients. Toss to coat and cook an additional 2 minutes.

3. Serve hot.

▶ SERVES 4

1 teaspoon paprika

½ teaspoon sea salt

½ teaspoon chili powder

1 teaspoon dried thyme

1 pound organic lamb steak

3 teaspoons olive oil, divided

1 teaspoon ghee

1 cup diced onions

8 ounces cremini mushrooms, diced

2 cups diced maitake mushrooms

1 tablespoon fresh thyme

1. Combine paprika, sea salt, chili powder, and dried thyme. Dice lamb steak into 2-inch pieces and sprinkle spice mixture evenly over the lamb, rubbing in with your hands to evenly distribute spices.

2. In a large sauté pan, heat 2 teaspoons olive oil over medium heat. Sear lamb 3 minutes per side so that the sides are crispy brown and the middle is light pink. Remove from pan and set aside.

3. In the same skillet, add remaining 1 teaspoon olive oil, ghee, and onion. Sauté 3 to 4 minutes, add mushrooms and fresh thyme, and sauté an additional 8 to 10 minutes until the mushrooms are soft and aromatic. Return lamb to the pan with mushrooms, tossing to combine.

4. Serve immediately.

▶ SERVES 4

Grilled Lamb Chops with Mint Pesto

1. Season lamb with salt, place in a sealable glass container. Pour olive oil over lamb, and sprinkle with garlic. Refrigerate at least an hour. Remove from fridge and let come to room temperature.

2. In a food processor, combine all pesto ingredients and pulse until smooth. Spoon into a small bowl and set aside.

3. Heat a grill pan over medium heat, and brush with olive oil. Grill lamb 6 to 7 minutes on each side for medium doneness.

4. Top with pesto and serve alongside Forbidden Black Rice Risotto*.

*See Forbidden Black Rice Risotto **NS** (page 147).

▶ SERVES 4

1 pound lamb chops
Sea salt, to taste
½ cup olive oil
3 cloves garlic, chopped

pesto:
½ cup fresh spinach
1 bunch fresh mint
1 teaspoon minced garlic
¼ cup extra virgin olive oil
½ teaspoon sea salt
Juice of 1 lemon
¼ cup raw walnuts

Lamb Moussaka–Stuffed Eggplant

2 medium eggplants

1 tablespoon plus 1 teaspoon olive oil, divided

Sea salt, to taste

1 cup diced onion

¼ cup raisins

2 cloves garlic, minced

½ teaspoon cumin

½ teaspoon ground ginger

1 jalapeno, seeded and finely diced

1 pound lean ground lamb

¼ cup ricotta cheese

1 cup bread crumbs*

1. Preheat oven to 400 degrees.

2. Slice eggplants lengthwise, and spoon out flesh and seeds to create an eggplant boat. Roughly chop insides and reserve. Set eggplant on a baking sheet, skin side down, and drizzle with 1 tablespoon olive oil and a pinch of sea salt. Bake for 30 minutes, remove from oven, and set aside.

3. In the meantime, heat remaining 1 teaspoon olive oil in skillet over medium heat. Add onion and raisins, and sauté about 4 minutes, just until raisins are plump and juicy and onions are opaque. Add reserved eggplant and sauté an additional 5 minutes, until eggplant is soft. Remove from pan and set aside.

4. In a small bowl, combine garlic, cumin, ginger, and jalapeno. Toss ground lamb with spice mixture and add to skillet. Brown lamb for 5 minutes, breaking up large pieces with a wooden spoon. Add onion and eggplant mixture back to the skillet and toss to combine. Remove from heat and stir in ricotta cheese.

5. Spoon lamb mixture into roasted eggplant boats, sprinkle with bread crumbs, and bake an additional 20 minutes. Eggplant boats will be tender and browned slightly on the bottom, filling will be warmed through, and bread crumbs will be golden brown. Serve warm.

*See Basic Bread Crumbs **NS** recipe (page 211).

▶ SERVES 4

Moroccan Lamb Tagine

2 teaspoons minced garlic

2 teaspoons minced ginger

¼ teaspoon ground cumin

½ teaspoon turmeric

8 ounces lamb fillet

2 teaspoons olive oil, divided

10 cippolini onions, peeled

1 cup chopped carrots

1 cup chopped parsnips

½ cup Vegetable Stock*

1 tablespoon lemon juice

1. In a small bowl, combine garlic, ginger, cumin, and turmeric. Rub spices on lamb fillets. Heat tagine over medium high heat, and brush with 1 teaspoon olive oil. When the tagine is hot, sear lamb in tagine just until browned on both sides. Remove from tagine and set aside.

2. To the tagine, add remaining 1 teaspoon olive oil, onions, carrots, and parsnips, and let cook 5 to 6 minutes.

3. Reduce heat to low. Place pieces of lamb on top of vegetables and add stock and lemon juice. Cover tagine and let cook for 1½ hours (no peeking). After 1½ hours, uncover. Most of the liquid should be absorbed, and lamb and vegetables will be tender. Serve warm.

*See Vegetable Stock **NS** recipe (page 211).

▶ SERVES 4

tip: A tagine is a Moroccan cooking vessel that has a heavy cast-iron or clay base and a domed, pyramid-shaped top, which creates a slow cooking method that adds moisture to each dish. As an alternative, try a cast-iron skillet and cover with tented tinfoil. Just make sure to seal the top of the skillet.

Sweet Potato Shepherd's Pie NS

2½ teaspoons olive oil, divided

3 cloves garlic, divided

Sea salt, to taste

4 cups sweet potato

1 tablespoon chopped fresh sage

1 tablespoon ghee or butter, divided

6 tablespoons 2 percent cow's milk

1 pound ground lamb

2 teaspoons paprika

2 tablespoons flour (brown rice, spelt, or oat)

1½ cups Beef Stock*

2 cups pearl onions

1 cup peas

2 cups finely diced carrots

1 cup shredded low-moisture mozzarella cheese

1. Preheat oven to 375 degrees.

2. Drizzle ½ teaspoon olive oil over two cloves of garlic and season with sea salt. Wrap in tinfoil and roast for 25 minutes.

3. While the garlic roasts, dice sweet potatoes into 2-inch pieces, and place in a medium pot with just enough water to cover. Bring to a boil and cook about 12 to 15 minutes, just until tender. Using a hand mixer, beat sweet potatoes with roasted garlic, sage, ghee, and milk. Season with sea salt, to taste.

4. Reduce oven temperature to 350 degrees.

5. Heat remaining 2 teaspoons olive oil in a large skillet over medium heat. Brown ground lamb for about 5 minutes, breaking up meat using a flat wooden spoon. Once browned, add paprika, and flour, stirring to coat. Add stock. Bring to a simmer, reduce heat, and cook 5 minutes, until sauce thickens.

6. Add onions, peas, and carrots to the skillet and stir to combine. Pour into a 9" x 11" baking dish, top with sweet potato mixture, spreading evenly with an offset spatula. Sprinkle on cheese and bake for 30 to 35 minutes, until the pie is hot and the cheese is melted and bubbling.

7. Serve warm.

*See Beef Stock **NS** recipe (page 212).

▶ SERVES 6

tip: As a time saver, frozen pearl onions can be used in this recipe instead of fresh.

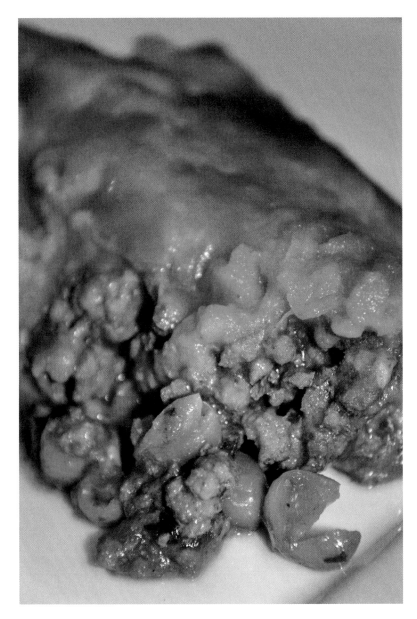

Tangy Pineapple and Beef Kabobs (NS)

Bamboo skewers, for grilling

marinade:

2 tablespoons fresh lemon juice

1 tablespoon agave

3 tablespoons olive oil

1 tablespoon fresh ginger, minced

½ teaspoon sweet paprika

1 teaspoon garlic, minced

kabobs:

1 pound organic beef tips

4 cups pineapple pieces

1 red onion, cut into ½-inch dice

1. Soak bamboo skewers in water for up to 1 hour before use to prevent burning.

2. Whisk together marinade ingredients in a bowl and set aside.

3. Trim any excess fat off beef. Place in a sealable glass dish, and pour ⅔ marinade over the beef, tossing to make sure all sides are coated with the marinade. Cover and place in the refrigerator for 3 hours.

4. Preheat grill or grill pan.

5. Alternate steak, pineapple, and onion, and repeat twice on each skewer. Brush pineapple and onion with marinade. Grill for 10 to 12 minutes, flipping halfway through cooking and brushing again with any remaining marinade.

6. Serve warm.

▶ SERVES 4

EAT RIGHT FOR YOUR TYPE PERSONALIZED COOKBOOK

1. Turn slow cooker to low.

2. Heat 1 teaspoons olive oil in a large skillet over medium heat, and sauté onion and carrots for 3 to 4 minutes. Remove vegetables from pan and place in slow cooker.

3. Combine spices in a small bowl, stirring to combine. Sprinkle spices over roast and gently massage into all sides.

4. Increase skillet heat to medium to medium-high. Add remaining 1 teaspoon olive oil and brown roast on all sides, cooking 1 to 2 minutes per side.

5. Remove roast from skillet and place in slow cooker. Pour stock and red wine into skillet to deglaze the pan, and use a flat spatula to loosen any bits stuck to bottom of the pan. Pour mixture over roast in slow cooker. Cover and cook on low for 5 hours.

6. Serve warm with Brown Rice Salad **NS** (page 146).

*See Beef Stock **NS** recipe (page 212).

▶ SERVES 4

2 teaspoons olive oil plus 1 teaspoon, divided

1 cup chopped onion

1 cup chopped carrots

1 teaspoon sea salt

½ teaspoon paprika

2 teaspoons dried parsley

1 teaspoon garlic powder

12 ounces venison roast

1 cup Beef Stock*

¼ cup red wine

Red Quinoa–Mushroom Casserole with Fried Egg NS

1 cup red quinoa

2 cups water

2 teaspoons ghee

½ cup diced shiitake mushrooms

1 cup diced maitake mushrooms

1½ cups diced okra

½ cup finely diced shallots

½ teaspoon mustard powder

½ teaspoon dry ginger

2 cloves garlic, minced

2 tablespoons fresh oregano

¾ cup finely diced pineapple

1 cup Vegetable Stock*

5 eggs, divided

1. Preheat oven to 350 degrees. Grease a 9" x 11" baking dish with nonstick olive oil spray and set aside.

2. Combine quinoa and water in a saucepan. Bring to a boil, reduce heat, and simmer for 12 minutes. Remove from heat, fluff with a fork, and set aside.

3. Heat a large skillet over medium heat, and melt ghee. Add mushrooms, okra, and shallots, and sauté 6 to 7 minutes. Remove from heat and set aside.

4. In a small bowl, whisk together mustard powder, ginger, garlic, oregano, pineapple, stock, and 1 egg. Set aside.

5. Toss quinoa with mushroom mixture, and place into prepared baking dish. Pour egg mixture evenly over casserole, and use a fork to make sure the liquid reaches all corners of the casserole.

6. Bake for 35 minutes, until casserole sets and becomes firm.

7. Just before removing casserole, fry remaining eggs in a skillet coated with nonstick cooking spray. Serve on top of warm casserole.

*See Vegetable Stock **NS** recipe (page 211).

▶ SERVES 6

EAT RIGHT FOR YOUR TYPE PERSONALIZED COOKBOOK

featured ingredient

red quinoa

Red quinoa is almost identical in nutritional content to regular quinoa, and it is a terrific source of fiber and protein, as it contains all nine essential amino acids. It also has a similar texture: light and fluffy with a slight crunch. The difference is that red quinoa has an earthier and less bitter taste. Use red quinoa in savory recipes, adding hearty vegetables, allowable cheeses, or beans.

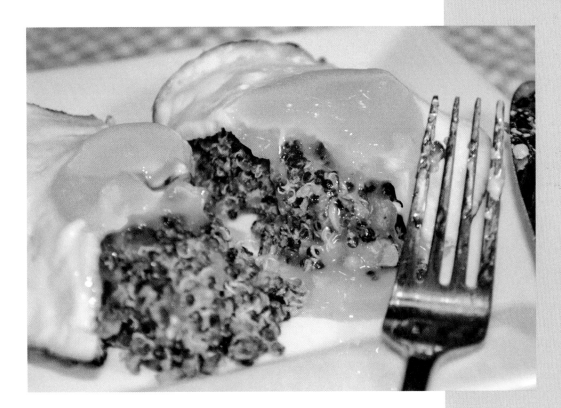

Greek Lamb Burgers NS

1 pound organic, free-range ground lamb

½ onion, grated

1 teaspoon minced garlic

1 tablespoon fresh oregano

½ teaspoon sea salt

1 teaspoon ghee or butter

2 cups diced cremini mushrooms

½ cup crumbled feta cheese

1. Place ground lamb in a large bowl. Add grated onion, garlic, oregano, and salt. Use your fingers to combine, but try not to overwork the meat or it will become tough. Shape into 6 patties.

2. Heat a skillet sprayed with olive oil spray over medium heat. Add burgers and cook 3 to 4 minutes per side, until crunchy brown on each side and tender, light pink in the center.

3. In a small skillet, heat ghee over medium heat. Sauté mushrooms until browned and tender, and season with sea salt, to taste. Top burgers with mushrooms and feta cheese. Serve warm on brown rice, millet, or spelt buns.

▶ SERVES 6

EAT RIGHT FOR YOUR TYPE PERSONALIZED COOKBOOK

1. Heat olive oil in a large pot over medium heat. Add eggplant, jalapenos, bell peppers, onion, and garlic, and sauté 4 to 5 minutes, until vegetables begin to soften and become aromatic. Remove vegetables from the pot and set aside.

2. Add meat to the same pot and break apart with a flat spoon or spatula. Once the meat is cooked and crumbled, add vegetables back to the pot and reduce heat to low.

3. Puree spinach in a food processor or blender with stock to create a smooth sauce.

4. Add pureed spinach and remaining ingredients to chili. Cover and let simmer at least 45 minutes, stirring occasionally to prevent burning.

5. Serve warm.

*See Vegetable Stock **NS** recipe (page 211).

▶ SERVES 4

2 teaspoons olive oil

1 cup diced eggplant

2 jalapenos, finely diced

1 cup diced green bell pepper

1 cup diced red bell pepper

2 cups chopped yellow onion

2 cloves garlic, minced

1 pound ground beef

5 cups spinach

½ cup Vegetable Stock*

2 teaspoons sweet paprika

1 teaspoon cumin

1 can navy beans, drained and rinsed

Navy Bean Stew NS

1 tablespoon olive oil

1 cup diced onions

¾ cup diced carrots

1 tablespoon diced serrano chilies

2 zucchini, diced

½ teaspoon cumin

3 cups navy beans, cooked and drained

5 cups Vegetable Stock*

½ teaspoon sea salt

1. Heat olive oil in a large Dutch oven over medium heat. Add onion, carrots, chilies, zucchini, and cumin, and sauté 6 to 7 minutes.

2. Add beans and Vegetable Stock, season with sea salt, to taste, and let cook a total of 30 to 35 minutes. Stew should be tender and steaming hot.

3. Serve warm.

*See Vegetable Stock NS recipe (page 211).

▶ SERVES 4

Bean Burgers

1. Place 1 cup of beans in a bowl and smash using a fork or potato masher.

2. In a large bowl, add mashed beans and all remaining ingredients, mixing gently just to combine. The mixture should be moist but easily held together. Form into 6 patties.

3. Heat a large skillet sprayed with olive oil spray over medium heat. Add the burgers and cook about 4 minutes per side. Serve warm with caramelized onions, toasted brown rice/millet buns, and crunchy lettuce.

*See Basic Bread Crumbs **NS** recipe (page 211).

▶ SERVES 6

2 cups cooked kidney beans, drained and rinsed, divided

1½ cups chopped baby spinach

¼ cup finely diced red bell pepper

½ cup shredded carrot

1 tablespoon plus 2 teaspoons olive oil

1 tablespoon fresh thyme

½ teaspoon sea salt

2 cloves garlic, minced

½ cup bread crumbs*

1 large egg, beaten

Olive oil spray

Type B 113

Spaghetti
Squash with
Creamy Goat
Cheese, Walnut,
and Parsley
Sauce **NS**

1. Preheat oven to 350 degrees.

2. Carefully halve squash from stem to base and scoop out seeds. Brush 2 teaspoons olive oil and sprinkle sea salt over flesh of squash. Roast, cut-side down, on a baking sheet for 35 to 40 minutes. Squash should be browned on the skin and flesh should be easily pierced with a fork. Remove and cool squash for 5 minutes.

3. Heat remaining 1 teaspoon olive oil in a small skillet over medium heat. Sauté onion 4 to 5 minutes, or until tender. Remove from heat and add goat cheese, walnuts, and parsley.

4. Take a fork and scrape insides of squash from stem to base. Squash will peel away from skin in long stands, resembling spaghetti. Place squash into a large bowl and toss with goat cheese sauce.

5. Serve warm.

▶ SERVES 4

1 large spaghetti squash

1 tablespoon olive oil, divided

½ teaspoon sea salt

¼ cup very finely diced onion

3 ounces goat cheese

1 cup toasted diced walnuts

1 cup finely diced parsley

Rice and Bean Loaf NS

½ cup brown rice, uncooked

2 cups shredded zucchini

½ cup diced onions

½ cup diced carrots

1 large egg, lightly beaten

2 cloves garlic, minced

½ cup bread crumbs*

¾ cup canned kidney beans, drained and rinsed

1 teaspoon paprika

½ cup navy beans, pureed

1. Preheat oven to 350 degrees. Spray a 8½" × 4½" loaf pan with nonstick cooking spray and set aside.

2. Combine rice with 1 cup water and cook according to package instructions. Let cool.

3. Spoon shredded zucchini onto a double layer of paper towels or cheese cloth and squeeze out excess liquid. Add zucchini to a large bowl with onions, carrots, cooked rice, egg, garlic, bread crumbs, kidney beans, and paprika. Toss to evenly distribute ingredients. Add pureed navy beans, stirring again to combine.

4. Place bean mixture in prepared loaf pan, using an offset spatula to spread evenly, and bake 25 to 30 minutes. The loaf should hold together and be firm but moist when done.

5. Serve warm.

*See Basic Bread Crumbs NS recipe (page 211).

▶ SERVES 4

Soups and Sides

Many times when preparing dinner, we think about eating a protein, vegetable, and complex carbohydrate, and although having them all together in one pot like chili or lasagna is ideal, it doesn't always work out that way. Therefore, it is essential to have a collection of quick, delicious side or soup options to pair with your protein choice. A number of vegetable- or complex carbohydrate–based soups and sides to keep on hand can be found in this section.

Thai Curry Soup (NS)

2–3 teaspoons olive oil

1 cup diced onion

1 teaspoon garlic, minced

1 tablespoon ginger, minced

⅛ teaspoon turmeric

¼ teaspoon curry powder

1 jalapeno, cut into ¼-inch rounds

1 green bell pepper, diced into ½-inch cubes

2 small turnips, diced

4 cups water

1 stick lemongrass

Sea salt, to taste

¼ cup 2 percent cow's milk

1 tablespoon sour cream

1. Heat olive oil in a stockpot over medium heat, Sauté onion, garlic, and ginger for 3 to 4 minutes until slightly tender and aromatic. Add turmeric, curry powder, jalapeno, bell peppers, and turnips. Stir and cook 5 minutes.

2. Pour water over vegetables. Bruise lemongrass by hitting it with the blunt edge of your knife to release the essential oils and then add lemongrass to the pot. Cover, and simmer for at least 30 minutes. Season with sea salt, to taste.

3. Whisk together milk and sour cream in a small bowl and set aside.

4. Remove lemongrass from soup just before serving. Pour cream mixture into soup, and stir to combine.

5. Serve warm.

▶ SERVES 6

featured ingredient

lemongrass

Lemongrass is a thick, woody stalk that needs to be bruised and chopped to bring out its flavor before being used in cooking. Lemongrass is most widely used in Asian cooking and adds a fresh, citrus flavor to dishes. Put into soups, rice, or quinoa for a great new twist on any recipe.

EAT RIGHT FOR YOUR TYPE PERSONALIZED COOKBOOK

Carrot-Ginger Soup NS

1. In a stockpot, heat olive oil and ghee over medium heat. Add onion, garlic, and carrots, sautéing 5 to 6 minutes until vegetables become tender. Add remaining ingredients and bring to a boil, reduce to a simmer, cover, and cook at least 30 minutes, or until carrots are fork-tender but not falling apart.

2. Puree soup with an immersion blender or standing blender until smooth. If the mixture appears too thick, add water until desired consistency is reached.

3. Serve warm.

▶ SERVES 6

1 teaspoon olive oil

2 teaspoons ghee

1 cup chopped onion

1 clove garlic

2 pounds carrots, peeled and diced

1 (3-inch) piece or about ¼ cup ginger, peeled and grated

½ teaspoon sea salt

1 tablespoon lemon zest

4 cups water

Roasted Parsnip Soup (NS)

4 cups diced parsnips

4 cups diced cauliflower

2 cloves garlic, peeled

2 tablespoons olive oil, divided

2 cups finely sliced sweet onion

Sea salt, to taste

2 Granny Smith apples, finely diced

1½ cups 2 percent cow's milk

1 cup water

⅛ teaspoon nutmeg

¼ cup chopped fresh sage

1. Preheat oven to 375 degrees.

2. Place parsnips, cauliflower, and garlic cloves on a sheet pan, and drizzle with 1 tablespoon olive oil and sprinkle with sea salt. Toss to coat.

3. Roast vegetables in the oven for 30 to 35 minutes, until tender and slightly golden brown around the edges.

4. About 15 minutes before the vegetables are finished cooking in the oven, heat remaining 1 tablespoon oil in a large stockpot over medium heat, and sauté onions for 8 to 10 minutes. Add apples, and sauté an additional 2 to 3 minutes.

5. Once the onions are tender and vegetables are done roasting, add roasted vegetables and remaining ingredients to stockpot. Bring the soup to a gentle boil, reduce heat, and simmer for 20 minutes. Blend with an immersion blender or puree in a standing blender until smooth and creamy.

6. Season with additional sea salt, to taste.

7. Serve warm.

▶ SERVES 6

Melted Mozzarella–Onion Soup NS

5 large white onions

1 tablespoon olive oil

½ tablespoon ghee or butter

½ cup red wine

4 sprigs thyme

2 sprigs sage

2 bay leaves

Sea salt, to taste

3 cups Beef Stock*

4 slices brown rice/millet bread, toasted

1 cup grated Gruyere cheese

1. Slice onions in half and then slice into thin, half-moon shapes.

2. In a large-bottomed stockpot, heat olive oil and ghee over medium heat. Add onions and caramelize for 12 minutes. Season with sea salt, reduce heat to medium-low, and cook an additional 20 minutes. Onions will become a rich, caramel color as the natural sugars in the onions release and sweeten them.

3. Add wine to the onions to deglaze the pan, and cook another 30 seconds. Add thyme, sage, bay leaves, salt, and stock. Bring to a boil, reduce heat, and simmer 30 minutes.

4. Spoon soup into 4 (7-oz.) high-sided, oven-safe bowls or ramekins. Top each with 1 slice toast then sprinkle with cheese, to create a cheesy bread lid for the soup.

5. Broil in oven for 2 minutes or until the cheese begins to bubble and brown slightly. Keep a close eye, as the toast and cheese can burn quickly.

6. Serve warm.

*See Beef Stock **NS** recipe (page 212).

▶ SERVES 4

Broccoli–Northern Bean Soup NS

1 tablespoon olive oil, divided

1 cup diced white onion

2 heads broccoli

1 clove garlic, minced

1 (15-oz.) can northern beans, drained and rinsed

2 cups Vegetable Stock*

4 sprigs fresh thyme

Sea salt, to taste

Pine nuts, to garnish

1. Heat 2 teaspoons olive oil in a stockpot over medium heat, add onion, and sauté 5 to 6 minutes.

2. Trim woody stems off broccoli and discard. Roughly chop the broccoli and remaining stems. Add to the onions along with garlic, beans, stock, and thyme. Bring to a boil, reduce heat, and simmer for 15 minutes. Vegetables should be tender and easily pierced with a fork, but not falling apart.

3. Puree soup using an immersion blender, or puree in batches in a regular blender, until smooth. Soup should be thick and creamy, but easily run off your spoon. Add water or additional stock if you prefer a thinner consistency. Season with sea salt, to taste.

4. Heat remaining 1 teaspoon olive oil in a small skillet over medium-low heat, and toast pine nuts for 2 to 3 minutes or until golden brown.

5. Serve soup hot and garnish with toasted pine nuts.

*See Vegetable Stock NS recipe (page 211).

▶ SERVES 6

EAT RIGHT FOR YOUR TYPE PERSONALIZED COOKBOOK

1. Heat 1 teaspoon olive oil in a Dutch oven over medium heat. Sauté ginger and garlic, stirring constantly to prevent burning.

2. Trim excess fat from beef and slice as thinly as possible. Add remaining 1 teaspoon olive oil to pot. Add meat and cook until browned, about 2 minutes.

3. Add cabbage, stock, water, onions, carrots, and bay leaf, and cook 30 minutes.

4. Add beans to the Dutch oven and cook until beans and carrots are tender, about 10 additional minutes. Remove bay leaf before serving and spoon soup into bowls.

5. Serve warm.

*See Beef Stock **NS** recipe (page 212).

▶ SERVES 4

2 teaspoons olive oil, divided

1 (1-inch) piece fresh ginger, peeled and minced

1 clove garlic, minced

¾ pound grass-fed, lean beef

Sea salt, to taste

2 cups shredded green cabbage

2 cups Beef Stock*

3 cups water

1 cup pearl onions

1 cup julienned carrots

1 bay leaf

2 cups haricots vert

Mushroom Soup with Parsley Pesto NS

1. Melt ghee in a stockpot over medium heat and add garlic and mushrooms. Sauté 3 to 4 minutes. Add stock and water, bring to boil, reduce heat to a simmer, and cook 5 minutes.

2. In the meantime, prepare pesto. In a food processor, combine parsley, garlic, olive oil, lemon juice, walnuts, and water. Season with sea salt, to taste.

3. Add quinoa to soup and simmer an additional 10 minutes. Add snow peas, cook 3 minutes, and serve with a dollop of pesto.

*See Vegetable Stock **NS** recipe (page 211).

▶ SERVES 6

soup:

2 teaspoons ghee

1 clove garlic

8 ounces cremini mushrooms, chopped

4 ounces shiitake mushrooms, chopped

4 cups Vegetable Stock*

3 cups water

¼ cup quinoa

¾ cup snow peas

pesto:

½ cup fresh parsley

1 clove garlic

2 tablespoons olive oil

2 tablespoons lemon juice

¼ cup raw walnuts

3 tablespoons water

Sea salt, to taste

Broccoli and Cabbage Slaw with Raisins (NS)

3 tablespoons lemon juice

3 tablespoons olive oil

2 teaspoons dry mustard

1 teaspoon honey or agave

Sea salt, to taste

½ small head of cabbage

2 heads broccoli

½ cup golden raisins

¼ cup chopped parsley

1. In a large bowl, whisk together lemon juice, olive oil, mustard, honey, and sea salt. Set aside.

2. Remove tough bottoms from cabbage as well as the outer layers. Grate the peeled cabbage into the bowl with the dressing. Cut bottoms and tops off broccoli stems, peel, and grate into same bowl with cabbage. A food processor can also be used for grating.

3. Add raisins and parsley, and toss to mix and coat with dressing.

4. Serve immediately or refrigerate and serve chilled.

▶ SERVES 4

tip: Reserve broccoli tops for a fast recipe: roast at 375 degrees with 2 teaspoons olive oil and a dash of sea salt for 20 minutes.

EAT RIGHT FOR YOUR TYPE PERSONALIZED COOKBOOK

1. Heat grill pan over medium heat.

2. Pull the leaves off the base of the bok choy and slice off the very bottom of the stem to remove any tough pieces. Wash the leaves individually and dry completely on a kitchen towel.

3. In a small bowl, whisk olive oil, ginger, garlic, and agave. Brush individual bok choy leaves with ginger mixture.

4. Grill leaves for about 30 to 45 seconds per side, until slightly wilted with golden-brown grill marks. Sprinkle with sea salt, to taste.

5. Serve warm.

▶ SERVES 4

1 (medium to large) bunch bok choy

2 teaspoons olive oil

1 tablespoon peeled, grated fresh ginger

1 teaspoon minced garlic

1 teaspoon agave

Sea salt, to taste

tip: When purchasing bok choy, look for stalks that are bright white in color with dark-colored greens. Avoid spotted stems and wilted leaves.

1. Heat ghee and olive oil in a large skillet over medium heat. Sauté shallots and turkey bacon until bacon is crispy, about 4 to 5 minutes.

2. Add Brussels sprouts, and continue to cook for 15 minutes, stirring occasionally to prevent burning. Add raisins and stock, and cook an additional 3 minutes so the raisins can become tender, and the broth can help deglaze the bottom of the pan and add moisture to the sprouts.

3. Sprouts are done when they can be pierced with a fork but still give moderate resistance. Be careful not to overcook, as they will become mushy and lose a lot of flavor.

4. Garnish with parsley and serve warm.

*See Vegetable Stock **NS** recipe (page 211).

▶ SERVES 4

1 teaspoon ghee

2 teaspoons olive oil

2 tablespoons finely diced shallots

4 strips nitrate- / preservative-free turkey bacon, diced

4 cups quartered Brussels sprouts

¼ cup golden raisins

½ cup Vegetable Stock*

1 tablespoon chopped parsley, for garnish

South Indian–Curried Eggplant (NS)

1 tablespoon olive oil

½ teaspoon mustard seeds

½ teaspoon cumin

½ teaspoon almonds

¾ cup finely diced onion

3 cups diced eggplant

1 cup diced red bell pepper

½ teaspoon turmeric

½ teaspoon sea salt

1 teaspoon red chili powder

1. Heat olive oil in a Dutch oven over medium heat. Add mustard seeds, cumin, and almonds, and cook 30 seconds. Add onions, and cook 5 minutes.

2. Add eggplant and bell peppers, and cook an additional 15 minutes. Add turmeric, salt, and chili powder, and let cook another 5 minutes.

3. Serve warm.

▶ SERVES 6

2 teaspoons olive oil

1 cup diced yellow onion

1 clove garlic, minced

1 teaspoon dry mustard

1 teaspoon molasses

1 teaspoon salt

1 teaspoon paprika

½ teaspoon chili powder

¼ teaspoon cayenne pepper

1 (6½-oz.) jar whole pimientos, drained

2 (15-oz.) cans navy beans, drained and rinsed

⅓ cup Vegetable Stock*

1. Preheat oven to 375 degrees.

2. Heat oil in Dutch oven over medium heat. Sauté onion and garlic until translucent and tender, about 5 to 7 minutes. Add mustard, molasses, salt, paprika, chili powder, and cayenne pepper, and cook 1 additional minute.

3. In a food processor or mini chopper, pulse pimientos until smooth.

4. Add navy beans, pimiento puree, and stock to pot. Stir to combine.

5. Cover and bake for 25 minutes until the beans are hot and the sauce is thick.

6. Serve warm.

*See Vegetable Stock **NS** recipe (page 211).

▶ SERVES 6

Spicy Collards NS

2 teaspoons olive oil

1 teaspoon ghee

½ cup diced shallots

4 slices nitrate- / preservative-free turkey bacon, finely diced

½ teaspoon chipotle chili powder

1 bunch collard greens

1 (15-oz.) can cannellini beans, drained and rinsed

Sea salt, to taste

1. Heat olive oil and ghee in a large skillet over medium heat. Add shallots and bacon, and sauté until bacon is crispy, about 4 to 5 minutes. Season with chili powder, add collard greens, and cook 10 to 12 minutes, until collards are tender and wilted.

2. Add beans, and cook an additional 3 to 4 minutes until warmed through.

3. Season with sea salt, to taste, and serve warm.

▶ SERVES 4

1. Preheat oven to 400 degrees.

2. Toss cauliflower florets with olive oil and sea salt and place on a baking sheet. Bake for 35 minutes, until softened and slightly browned on the bottoms. Remove from oven and set aside.

3. Melt ghee in a Dutch oven over medium heat. Sauté garlic and onion for 5 to 6 minutes. Add oat flour and stir for about 1 minute just to cook out the taste of the flour. Slowly add milk and stock, whisking continuously to avoid lumps. Continue whisking until mixture becomes the consistency of yogurt, about 5 minutes.

4. Add spinach, ¼ at a time, just so it has a chance to cook down and make room for the next batch.

5. Once all the spinach has been added, toss in roasted cauliflower. Serve warm.

*See Vegetable Stock NS recipe (page 211).

▶ SERVES 4

2 cups cauliflower florets

2 teaspoons olive oil

Sea salt, to taste

1 tablespoon ghee

2 cloves garlic, minced

1 cup finely diced white onion

3 tablespoons oat flour

½ cup 2 percent cow's milk

¾ cup Vegetable Stock*

10 cups roughly chopped baby spinach

1 celery root

1 turnip

2 carrots

2 cups cauliflower florets

4 shallots, diced

1 tablespoon olive oil

1 teaspoon sea salt

2 tablespoons chopped fresh sage

1. Preheat oven to 400 degrees.

2. Peel celery root, turnip, and carrots. Dice celery, turnip, and carrots into 2-inch pieces.

3. Toss vegetables, shallots, olive oil, sea salt, and sage in a large bowl until evenly coated.

4. Pour onto a baking sheet and bake for 55 to 60 minutes, until all vegetables are tender and browned around the edges.

5. Serve warm.

▶ SERVES 4

featured ingredient

celery root

Otherwise known as celeriac, celery root is just what it seems: the root of a type of celery. It has a deliciously fresh flavor that is a cross between celery and parsley, but works terrifically as a base for soups with onions and carrots, eaten raw, or roasted (as featured above). A *Neutral* for all blood types, this vegetable adds a diversity of flavor to your palate.

2 heads escarole,
washed and dried

2 teaspoons olive oil

¼ teaspoon large-grain
sea salt

1. Preheat oven to 375 degrees.

2. Trim woody stems off the bottom of escarole and discard, and give the leaves a rough chop. Toss with olive oil and season with sea salt.

3. Spread escarole evenly across two baking sheets. Bake 10 to 12 minutes, stirring once after 5 minutes. Escarole should be dark green and wilted with crispy, slightly browned edges.

4. Serve immediately.

▶ SERVES 4

1. Preheat oven to 375 degrees.

2. Prepare mustard greens by washing and patting dry with a kitchen towel. Remove greens from woody stems and roughly chop or tear into bite-size pieces. Toss with olive oil, sea salt, and cayenne pepper. Spread on a baking sheet and place on the top rack of the oven. Bake 12 minutes, until wilted and slightly crispy around the edges.

3. Transfer to a serving bowl and add crumbled feta.

4. Serve warm.

▶ SERVES 4

1 medium bunch mustard greens

2 teaspoons olive oil

½ teaspoon sea salt

¼ teaspoon cayenne pepper

½ cup crumbled feta cheese

Ratatouille

NS

1 medium eggplant

Sea salt, to taste

2 medium red bell peppers

1 bulb fennel

1 large white onion

1 tablespoon olive oil, divided

1 cup peas

½ cup chopped parsley

2 cloves garlic

½ cup grated hard goat cheese

1. Preheat oven to 375 degrees.

2. Slice eggplant in ¼-inch-thick rounds, set on a towel, and sprinkle with sea salt to draw out excess moisture. Slice red bell pepper, fennel, and onion in a similar fashion, set aside.

3. Heat 2 teaspoons olive oil in a large skillet over medium heat. When hot, carefully brown red bell pepper, fennel, and onion in a single layer on the bottom of the pan. Cook vegetables 2 to 3 minutes per side, just to brown. Remove from skillet and set aside.

4. Pat excess moisture off eggplant slices, and brown in the same skillet, cooking 2 to 3 minutes per side, adding additional oil if necessary. Remove from pan and set aside.

5. Return skillet to stovetop and increase heat to medium-high. Puree peas in a mini food processor. Add to pan with parsley and garlic, and sauté for 3 to 4 minutes.

6. In a baking dish, layer red bell pepper and eggplant across the bottom, top with pea mixture and ¼ cup goat cheese. Top with onion, fennel, and remaining cheese.

7. Bake uncovered for 20 minutes.

8. Serve warm or let come to room temperature or store in refrigerator, and serve cold.

▶ SERVES 4

Roasted Broccoli with Garlic-Basil Oil **NS**

1. Preheat oven to 375 degrees.

2. Dice broccoli into bite-size pieces, and toss with olive oil and sea salt. Place on a sheet pan or in a baking dish, and roast for 25 minutes. Broccoli will be deep green with slightly browned edges.

3. While the broccoli roasts, make basil oil by pureeing garlic, basil, lemon juice, olive oil, and water until thin and runny.

4. Serve broccoli drizzled with garlic-basil oil.

▶ SERVES 4

1 head broccoli
2 teaspoons olive oil
Sea salt, to taste

basil oil:

1 clove garlic
1 cup finely chopped basil
1 tablespoon lemon juice
1 tablespoon olive oil
1–2 tablespoons water

Roasted Sweet Potatoes with Fried Sage

2 large sweet potatoes

1 tablespoon plus 2 teaspoons olive oil

Sea salt, to taste

⅛ teaspoon nutmeg

2 tablespoons fresh sage

1. Preheat oven to 400 degrees.

2. Leaving skins on potatoes, cut off tough ends and slice in half lengthwise. Cut in ¼-inch-thick half-moon shapes and toss with 2 teaspoons olive oil, a dash of sea salt, and nutmeg. Place sweet potato slices in a single layer on a baking sheet, and roast for 25 to 30 minutes or until slightly browned and tender.

3. During last few minutes of cooking, heat remaining 1 tablespoon olive oil in a small skillet over medium heat. Place sage in pan and fry until crispy, no more than 30 seconds. Remove with a slotted spoon onto a paper towel. Important note: make sure sage is perfectly dry, as wetness on the leaves will splatter the hot oil.

4. Remove sweet potatoes from oven and serve garnished with crumbled fried sage.

▶ SERVES 4

EAT RIGHT FOR YOUR TYPE PERSONALIZED COOKBOOK

1. Preheat oven to 350 degrees. Grease bottom and sides of 8 (4-oz.) ramekins. Set aside.

2. In a small saucepan, gently warm milk with 2 sprigs of sage for 10 to 12 minutes.

3. While the milk heats, whisk together egg yolks, brown rice flour, and maple syrup. When milk is ready, temper egg yolks by very slowly pouring about ½ cup of warm milk into the egg mixture, stirring continuously. Pour the tempered eggs back into the saucepan with the remaining milk. Increase heat to medium, and stir until thickened, 2 to 3 minutes.

4. In a medium bowl, beat baked sweet potato with ghee, finely chopped sage, and salt. When milk mixture has thickened, remove from heat, and whisk in whipped sweet potato until smooth. Cool completely.

5. In a dry, glass, stainless steel, or copper bowl, beat egg whites until they form stiff peaks. Fold egg whites into cooled sweet potato mixture ⅓ at a time. Once the egg whites are completely incorporated, spoon batter into prepared ramekins, filling each ramekin ¾ of the way up the sides. Place ramekins in a high-sided baking dish, and place in oven with the oven rack extended out of the oven. Pour 1 inch of hot water into the bottom of the baking dish. Bake soufflés for 55 to 60 minutes or until firm.

6. Serve immediately.

▶ SERVES 6

1½ cups 2 percent cow's milk

2 sprigs fresh sage

3 egg yolks

¼ cup brown rice flour

1 tablespoon maple syrup

1 cup sweet potato, baked

1 tablespoon ghee or butter

1 tablespoon fresh sage, finely chopped

1 teaspoon sea salt

6 large egg whites

tip: Egg whites cannot be beaten in a bowl that holds fat, such as plastic. Rather, a glass, copper, or stainless steel bowl will enable to eggs to be beaten into stiff peaks. Water inside the bowl will also prohibit egg whites from stiffening, so make sure to carefully wipe down the inside of the bowl prior to use.

2 rutabaga roots

1 head broccoli

¼ cup roughly chopped parsley

¼ cup 2 percent cow's milk

2 cloves garlic, peeled

2 teaspoons ghee or butter

Sea salt, to taste

1. Peel rutabaga and dice in approximately 1-inch pieces to ensure even cooking. Place in a pot with cold, salted water and bring to a boil. Reduce heat, cover, simmer for 35 minutes, or until rutabaga is fork-tender.

2. Bring a second pot of water to a boil. Trim stems off broccoli and dice into bite-size pieces. Steam 5 to 6 minutes, until bright green and tender. Drain and set aside.

3. Drain rutabaga and return to pot. Use a potato masher or fork to mash rutabaga, and add parsley, milk, garlic, butter, and salt. Cook 3 to 4 minutes, until butter melts and flavors incorporate, and fold in broccoli.

4. Serve warm.

▶ SERVES 4

Sweet Potato Hash with Turkey Sausage

6 cups sliced sweet potatoes

2 teaspoons ghee

1 cup diced onion

1 cup diced green bell pepper

2 links raw turkey sausage

2 teaspoons olive oil

Sea salt, to taste

1 tablespoon maple syrup

1. Slice sweet potatoes into matchsticks, about 2 inches long and ¼-inch thick. Place sweet potatoes in a large pot of cold water and bring to a boil. As soon as the water boils, drain and spread sweet potatoes out on a baking sheet lined with a kitchen towel, set aside to dry.

2. Heat 2 teaspoons ghee in a large skillet over medium heat. Sauté onion and bell pepper for 3 to 4 minutes, until tender. Remove turkey sausage from casings and add to onion. Cook for 5 minutes, breaking apart with a flat spatula.

3. Remove sausage and vegetables from pan and set aside. Add olive oil to skillet, and add sweet potatoes. Do not stir for 2 minutes so potatoes brown on one side. Flip, and let cook undisturbed for 2 to 3 minutes to brown the opposite side. Add sausage and vegetables to the pan with maple syrup and stir gently, just to combine.

4. Serve hot.

▶ SERVES 6

1 small onion

2 medium carrots

2 stalks celery

1 large parsnip

2 teaspoons olive oil

1 clove garlic, minced

¾ cup organic sweet potato puree

3 tablespoons chopped sage, divided

½ cup Vegetable Stock*

Sea salt, to taste

1 cup Rice Polenta*

1. Peel and dice onions, carrots, celery, and parsnips into ¼- to ½-inch dice.

2. Heat olive oil in a large sauté pan over medium heat. Sauté vegetables 5 to 6 minutes until vegetables begin to soften.

3. Add garlic, sweet potato puree, 2 tablespoons sage, and stock. Season with sea salt, to taste.

4. Bring to a boil, reduce heat to low, and cook for 20 to 30 minutes, stirring occasionally. Finished ragu should be creamy, and all vegetables should be fork-tender.

5. Serve warm on top of Rice Polenta, and garnish with remaining sage.

*See Vegetable Stock **NS** recipe (page 211). See Creamy Rice Polenta **NS** recipe (page 152).

▶ SERVES 4

Brown Rice Salad

¾ cup brown rice

1½ cups water

2 teaspoons olive oil

½ cup diced celery

1 tablespoon chopped fresh sage

1 cup diced shiitake mushrooms

1 cup diced silver dollar mushrooms

¼ cup finely diced shallots

2 cups arugula

2 tablespoons toasted almonds

1. Cook brown rice in water according to package instructions. Remove from heat and set aside to cool slightly.

2. Heat olive oil in a medium skillet over medium heat, and sauté celery, sage, mushrooms, and shallots for 3 to 4 minutes, until vegetables just begin to soften.

3. In a large serving bowl, toss brown rice, sautéed mushroom mixture, arugula, and toasted almonds. The brown rice will be warm and will wilt the arugula slightly.

4. Serve warm or room temperature.

▶ SERVES 4

Forbidden Black Rice Risotto **NS**

1. Heat stock and milk in a small pot over low heat.

2. Heat olive oil in a Dutch oven over medium heat. Sauté onion and rice for 3 to 4 minutes, stirring constantly.

3. Add stock mixture, one ladle at a time, to the rice and onions. Season with sea salt. When the liquid is absorbed, add the next ladle. Repeat until all the liquid has been used; this process will take about 45 minutes.

4. Serve warm.

*See Vegetable Stock **NS** recipe (page 211).

▶ SERVES 4

2 teaspoons olive oil

½ cup finely diced white onion

1 cup forbidden black rice

2 cups Vegetable Stock*

¾ cup 2 percent cow's milk

½ teaspoon sea salt

Herbed Quinoa **NS**

1 cup quinoa

1 cup Vegetable Stock*

1 cup water

1 tablespoon fresh rosemary

1 tablespoon fresh thyme

1 tablespoon fresh parsley

½ teaspoon lemon zest

2 tablespoons flaxseeds

¼ cup crumbled feta cheese

1. Combine quinoa, stock, and water in a pot. Bring to a boil, reduce heat, and simmer for 10 to 12 minutes. When quinoa is done, all the water will be absorbed, and quinoa will be soft and tender.

2. Fluff cooked quinoa with a fork, and toss with remaining ingredients. Serve warm.

*See Vegetable Stock **NS** recipe (page 211).

▶ SERVES 4

1 small head broccoli

1 bunch broccolini

1 (4-inch) piece lemongrass

1 cup quinoa

2 cups water

2 teaspoons olive oil

1 red bell pepper, diced

1 tablespoon lemon zest

Sea salt, to taste

1. Bring a large pot of water to a boil. Chop broccoli and broccolini into bite-size pieces, drop into water, and cook for 3 minutes. Remove with a slotted spoon, and place in an ice bath to stop the cooking process. Drain and set aside on a kitchen towel.

2. Bruise lemongrass by hammering with the back of your knife, just until aromatic. Bring quinoa and water to a boil with a pinch of salt, and reduce heat to simmer. Add lemongrass to the quinoa, and let cook 12 minutes.

3. Heat olive oil in a large skillet over medium heat, and sauté bell pepper for 3 to 4 minutes. Add broccoli and broccolini, and sauté an additional 2 to 3 minutes. Vegetables should be crisp-tender and remain brightly colored when finished cooking. Remove lemongrass from cooked quinoa. Toss vegetables with quinoa and lemon zest, adding sea salt, to taste.

4. Serve warm or cold.

▶ SERVES 6

Mint and Red Pepper Tabbouleh NS

2 cups diced red bell pepper

3 tablespoons plus 2 teaspoons olive oil, divided

Sea salt, to taste

4 cups torn kale

1 cup raw quinoa

2 cups water

1 tablespoon lemon juice

1 tablespoon lemon zest

2 cloves garlic, minced

2 cups parsley leaves

¾ cup mint leaves

1. Preheat oven to 400 degrees.

2. Dice peppers into ½-inch pieces, and toss with 2 teaspoons olive oil and a dash of sea salt. Place in a single layer on a baking sheet and bake 10 minutes.

3. In the meantime, drizzle 2 teaspoons olive oil over kale on a baking sheet and sprinkle with sea salt. After the peppers have cooked for 10 minutes, put the kale in the oven as well. Bake for an additional 12 minutes, until kale pieces are crispy and peppers are tender. Remove vegetables from oven and set aside.

4. Combine quinoa and water with a dash of sea salt. Bring to a boil, cover, reduce heat, and simmer for 10 minutes. Remove from heat and let sit, covered, for an additional 4 to 5 minutes. Fluff with a fork and set aside to cool.

5. Whisk remaining olive oil, lemon juice and zest, and garlic in the bottom of a large bowl. Toss with parsley, mint, peppers, cooked quinoa, and kale until dressing is evenly distributed.

6. Serve room temperature or chilled.

▶ SERVES 6

2 large white potatoes (NS substitute sweet potatoes)

½ cup 2 percent cow's milk

1 tablespoon butter

2 tablespoons fresh chopped rosemary

¼ cup water

½ cup chopped walnuts

Sea salt, to taste

1 cup shredded mozzarella or Gruyere cheese

1. Preheat oven to 375 degrees.

2. Scrub potatoes, and thinly slice into ¼-inch-thick rounds. Place in a bowl of cold water and set aside.

3. In a small saucepan, bring milk, butter, rosemary, and water to a simmer over medium heat.

4. In a food processor, pulse walnuts until crumbled. Gradually drizzle in half of the hot milk mixture, and puree until the mixture is as thick as a heavy cream. Add sea salt, to taste.

5. Drain potatoes from water, and set on a kitchen towel to dry. Spoon a small amount of walnut cream in the bottom of 4 (12-oz.) ramekins. Top with a layer of potato, followed by walnut cream and shredded cheese. Repeat until the layers of potato have reached the top of the ramekins, and finish with cream and cheese. Pour remaining milk mixture evenly over each ramekin, and bake for 30 to 35 minutes until hot and bubbling.

6. Serve warm.

▶ SERVES 4

Creamy Rice Polenta **NS**

½ cup brown rice farina

1 teaspoon dry parsley

¼ cup mozzarella cheese

2 teaspoons olive oil

½ teaspoon onion powder

1. Cook brown rice farina according to package instructions. Two minutes before farina is finished cooking, add remaining ingredients, stirring constantly.

2. Serve immediately.

▶ SERVES 2

tip: If farina is ready before the rest of your meal and becomes too thick, simply add warm water 1 tablespoon at a time until desired consistency is achieved.

Snacks

Cheese Toast **NS** ▪ Summer Squash Salsa **NS** ▪ Crudités and Creamy Goat Cheese Dip **NS** ▪ Navy Bean Hummus **NS** ▪ Flax Crackers **NS** ▪ Curried Egg Salad **NS** ▪ Farmer Cheese and Beet-Endive Cups **NS** ▪ Marinated Mozzarella Balls **NS** ▪ Spicy Rosemary-Nut Mix **NS** ▪ Broccolini with Crispy Walnut Bacon **NS** ▪ Crispy Spring Vegetable Cakes **NS** ▪ Roasted Cauliflower Bruschetta **NS** ▪ Homemade Applesauce ▪ Tropical Fruit Salad with Mint and Lime Dressing **NS** ▪ Pear and Apple Chips ▪ Baked Grapefruit ▪ Grilled Pineapple with Chocolate Syrup ▪ Almond-Butter Rice Cakes with Mini Chips **NS** ▪ Carob–Walnut Butter–Stuffed Figs **NS**

Snacks **tend to** be the most difficult place for most people to get creative and come up with new ideas that are not overly complicated. Hopefully you will come across a few new options that will make snacking easier, tastier, and healthier. There are also a few snacks that translate well as appetizers if you like entertaining or have a little extra time to prepare something special.

Cheese Toast NS

2 slices spelt bread

1 clove garlic, halved

2 teaspoons olive oil

2 thin slices fresh mozzarella cheese

½ teaspoon dried oregano

1 tablespoon chopped fresh basil

1. Preheat broiler to highest setting.

2. Lightly toast bread, and rub halved garlic, cut-side down, on toast. Drizzle with olive oil, top with mozzarella cheese, and garnish with oregano.

3. Place under broiler for 1 to 2 minutes or until cheese is melted and bubbling. Keep an eye on the toast so the cheese does not burn.

4. Garnish with basil. Serve warm.

▶ SERVES 2

1. Heat olive oil in a 2-quart pot over medium heat. Sauté onion and garlic for 8 to 10 minutes.

2. Dice parsnips and summer squash into ½-inch cubes. Add to onions and garlic and sauté until tender, about 10 minutes.

3. Add butternut squash puree, stock, and sage. Bring to a gentle boil, reduce heat, and simmer 5 minutes.

4. Season with sea salt and serve as a warm salsa or let cool in refrigerator and serve chilled.

*See Vegetable Stock NS recipe (page 211).

▶ SERVES 4

2 teaspoons olive oil

1 cup diced sweet onion

1 large garlic clove, minced

1 large parsnip, peeled

2 medium summer squash

1 cup butternut squash puree

½ cup Vegetable Stock*

1 tablespoon chopped fresh sage

Sea salt, to taste

Crudités and Creamy Goat Cheese Dip

dip:

4 ounces soft goat cheese

2 tablespoons chopped dill

2 teaspoons agave

½ teaspoon sea salt

1 tablespoon lemon juice

1 tablespoon nonfat cow's milk

crudites:

Baby carrots

Raw broccoli florets

Red and orange bell peppers

1. Whisk all dip ingredients in a bowl until smooth and seasonings are fully incorporated.

2. Spoon into a serving dish, and plate with vegetables.

▶ SERVES 4

EAT RIGHT FOR YOUR TYPE PERSONALIZED COOKBOOK

Navy Bean Hummus

1. Put all ingredients in a food processor or a mini chopper and puree until smooth and creamy.

2. Serve with Flax Crackers* or crudités.

*See Flax Crackers **NS** recipe (page 159).

▶ SERVES 4

1½ cups navy beans, cooked and drained

½ cup chopped fresh basil

2 tablespoons chopped fresh parsley

1 clove garlic, minced

2 teaspoons olive oil

1 tablespoon walnuts

1 teaspoon lemon zest

1. Combine flaxseeds with water, stir, and set aside for 15 minutes.

2. Preheat oven to 200 degrees.

3. The flax mixture will become thick and goopy. Add remaining ingredients, stirring to combine. Batter will be slightly thicker and should hold together well at this point.

4. Cover a baking sheet with parchment paper and pour flax mixture onto the center of the sheet. Spray an offset spatula with cooking spray or coat with olive oil to help you spread the flax mixture without sticking. Try to spread the mixture in a thin layer as evenly as possible across the whole baking sheet.

5. Bake for 2 hours, flipping once halfway through. Once baked, crackers will be stiff and crunchy. Remove from oven and let cool a few moments before breaking into pieces. Serve warm or room temperature.

6. Once fully cooled, store in a cool, dry place for 2 to 3 days, or in the freezer for up to 1 month.

▶ SERVES 4

1 cup ground flaxseeds
⅔ cup hot water
¼ teaspoon sea salt
½ cup finely ground walnuts
Nonstick cooking spray

1. Place eggs in a saucepan, and cover with cold water. Bring to a boil, and turn off the heat. Set a timer for 14 minutes, and when done, rinse eggs under cold water. Peel eggs, chop, and place them in a large bowl.

2. Add remaining ingredients to the bowl, and toss to combine.

3. Serve on celery sticks or between two pieces of brown-rice toast.

▶ SERVES 4

4 large eggs

½ teaspoon dried mustard

1 tablespoon chopped fresh parsley

¼ teaspoon sea salt

½ teaspoon curry powder

⅛ teaspoon turmeric

2 teaspoons olive oil

2 teaspoons lemon juice

Farmer Cheese and Beet-Endive Cups NS

2 medium orange beets
2 medium red beets
2 teaspoons olive oil
¼ cup farmer cheese
¼ cup chopped walnuts
1 teaspoon lemon juice
Sea salt, to taste
2 heads of endive

1. Preheat oven to 400 degrees. Line a baking sheet with tinfoil and set aside.

2. Trim tops and bottoms off orange and red beets, and scrub clean. Drizzle beets with olive oil and roast for 60 to 65 minutes or until easily pierced with a knife.

3. Let beets cool for 10 minutes, then carefully remove skin with a paring knife and dice into ½-inch cubes. Toss into a bowl with farmer cheese, walnuts, and lemon juice. Season to taste with sea salt.

4. Wash, dry, and separate endive leaves. Spoon about 2 teaspoons of filling onto each endive leaf.

5. Serve immediately or chill, covered, in the refrigerator until ready to serve.

▶ SERVES 4

tip: Store-bought precooked beets—either canned or in vacuum-sealed packages in the produce department—can be used in this recipe, but beets from a can tend to lose a great deal of flavor and sweetness.

½ cup extra virgin olive oil

1 teaspoon large-grain sea salt

1 teaspoon crushed red pepper flakes

2 cloves garlic, minced

2 tablespoons chopped basil

1 pound fresh mozzarella balls

1. Whisk oil, salt, pepper flakes, garlic, and basil in a medium-size bowl so that everything is incorporated. Add mozzarella balls, toss to coat, and refrigerate for at least 2 hours.

2. Remove from refrigerator 15 minutes before serving, to allow oil to come to room temperature.

3. Mozzarella balls will keep in the refrigerator for up to 1 week.

▶ SERVES 4

tip: If you cannot find individually portioned miniature mozzarella balls, buy one large ball of fresh cheese and cut into 1- to 2-inch pieces as a substitute.

Spicy Rosemary-Nut Mix **NS**

2 tablespoons fresh rosemary

1 teaspoon red chili powder

½ teaspoon salt

1 tablespoon maple syrup

2 teaspoons ghee

1 cup black walnuts, quartered

½ cup chopped macadamia nuts

½ cup crushed almonds

1. Preheat oven to 325 degrees.

2. Toss all ingredients in a bowl and spread on a baking sheet. Bake for 25 minutes, tossing once halfway through. When cooked, nuts will be aromatic and lightly browned. Let cool and spoon into a bowl to serve.

3. Store in a cool, dry place for up to 1 week.

▶ SERVES 6

Broccolini with Crispy Walnut Bacon (NS)

1. Preheat oven to 375 degrees.

2. In a small bowl, combine maple syrup, ginger, and walnuts. Set aside.

3. Prepare broccolini by cutting off woody ends and separating into individual spears. Toss with olive oil.

4. Slice bacon lengthwise and then into thirds. Wrap bacon around each spear of broccolini, and place on a wire rack. Repeat until all broccolini is wrapped.

5. Place wire rack on a baking sheet. Spoon the maple-walnut mixture over bacon.

6. Bake for 10 to 12 minutes on middle rack until walnuts are toasty brown, bacon is cooked and crispy, and broccolini is bright green with slightly browned bottoms.

7. Serve warm.

▶ SERVES 6

2 tablespoons maple syrup

1 teaspoon ground ginger

½ cup finely chopped walnuts

2 bunches broccolini

2 teaspoons olive oil

5 slices nitrate- / preservative-free turkey bacon

1. Place celeriac, fennel, and onion in a bowl. Add kale, lemon zest, sage, egg, flour, and bread crumbs. Toss to combine.

2. Heat oil in a skillet over medium heat. Use a 1¾-inch ice cream scoop for perfect-size portions (you can also use a ¼-cup measurer if you do not have an ice cream scoop), spooning vegetable-cake mixture into the pan about 1 to 2 inches apart from each other for even cooking. Let cook 2 to 3 minutes, flip, and cook an additional 2 to 3 minutes on the other side.

3. Serve immediately.

*See Basic Bread Crumbs NS recipe (page 211).

▶ SERVES 4

1 cup grated celeriac (celery root)

1 cup grated fennel

2 tablespoons grated onion

2 cups finely chopped kale

½ teaspoon lemon zest

1 tablespoon chopped sage

1 large egg

2 tablespoons brown rice flour

⅓ cup bread crumbs*

2 teaspoons olive oil

tip: Cool and refrigerate cakes to eat for a snack or breakfast topped with a poached or fried egg.

Roasted Cauliflower Bruschetta

NS

1½ cups cauliflower florets

2 cloves peeled garlic

1 tablespoon olive oil, divided

Sea salt, to taste

2 cups chopped spinach

¼ cup crumbled feta cheese

3 slices brown rice or spelt bread, toasted

1. Preheat oven to 400 degrees.

2. Spread cauliflower and garlic in a single layer on a sheet pan. Drizzle with olive oil and sea salt (do not salt too heavily because feta cheese is salty). Roast for 30 minutes, until cauliflower is soft and golden brown around the edges.

3. Toss hot cauliflower with spinach in a bowl to wilt the spinach slightly. Rub roasted garlic on toast and slice toast in quarters.

4. Add feta cheese to cauliflower mixture and spoon evenly over toast to serve.

▶ SERVES 2

1. Peel apples and dice into 1-inch cubes.

2. Combine apples, apple juice, and cranberries in a saucepan over medium heat. Add 1 tablespoon agave to start, but depending on the tartness of the apples and cranberries, an additional tablespoon may be needed. Cook for 30 minutes or until apples no longer hold their shape.

3. Stir occasionally, remove from heat, and serve warm or chilled.

▶ SERVES 6

2 Red Delicious organic apples

2 Granny Smith organic apples

½ cup apple juice

½ cup (fresh or frozen) organic cranberries

1–2 tablespoons agave

½ cup dried cranberries

2 cups fresh cherries

1 papaya

1 pineapple

2 organic mangoes

Zest and juice of 2 limes

1 teaspoon agave

½ cup finely chopped mint leaves

1. Place dried cranberries in a small bowl. Cover with hot water and steep for 10 minutes, to rehydrate.

2. Peel and dice papaya, pineapple, and mango into ½-inch pieces and toss in a large serving bowl with fresh cherries.

3. Strain cranberries from water, and gently pat dry on a kitchen towel. Add to serving bowl.

4. Whisk lime zest, juice, agave, and mint leaves, and pour over fruit salad.

5. Toss and serve chilled.

▶ SERVES 6

Pear and Apple Chips

2 Bosc pears
2 Bartlett pears
2 Braeburn apples

1. Preheat oven to 225 degrees. Line 2 baking sheets with parchment paper and set aside.

2. Slice pears and apples in rounds as thinly as you can, or use a mandolin to help you. Line sliced fruit in a single layer on prepared baking sheets.

3. Bake for 2 hours, flipping fruit halfway through cooking.

4. Let cool completely and serve.

▶ SERVES 4

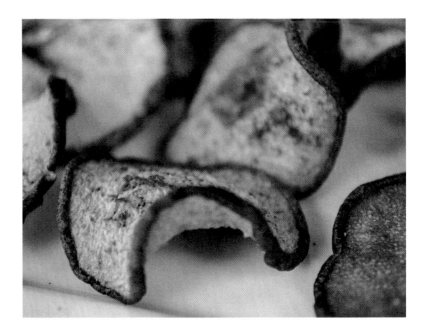

EAT RIGHT FOR YOUR TYPE PERSONALIZED COOKBOOK

Baked Grapefruit

1. Preheat oven to 400 degrees.

2. Trim the rounded bottom of each grapefruit half to create a stable base. Place on a baking sheet, flesh side up.

3. Drizzle each half evenly with honey.

4. Bake for 5 to 6 minutes, and then broil for 1 to 2 additional minutes, until the edges of the grapefruit are browned, the fruit is hot, and the topping is bubbling.

5. Serve warm.

▶ SERVES 4

2 ruby red grapefruits, halved

2 teaspoons honey

Grilled Pineapple with Chocolate Syrup

2 teaspoons light olive oil
1 fresh pineapple
¼ cup Chocolate Syrup*

1. Preheat a grill pan over medium heat. Brush with oil to create a nonstick surface.

2. Remove outer layer of pineapple, core, and slice into 1/2-inch-thick rounds.

3. Brush one side of pineapple rounds with chocolate syrup, and place syrup-side down on the grill pan. Let cook 2 to 3 minutes, and brush the opposite side with chocolate syrup.

4. Flip and grill an additional 2 to 3 minutes.

5. Serve warm.

*See Chocolate Syrup **NS** recipe (page 209).

▶ SERVES 4

EAT RIGHT FOR YOUR TYPE PERSONALIZED COOKBOOK

Almond-Butter Rice Cakes with Mini Chips (NS)

4 tablespoons almond butter

2 rice cakes

1 banana

2 tablespoons mini dark chocolate chips

1 teaspoon honey

1. Spread 2 tablespoons almond butter on each rice cake, and top each with slices from ½ banana, 1 tablespoon chocolate chips, and ½ teaspoon honey.

▶ SERVES 2

Carob–Walnut Butter–Stuffed Figs

NS

5 fresh or dried figs

¼ cup walnut halves

2 tablespoons pecans

1 tablespoon Carob Extract™ plus more for garnishing*

1 teaspoon olive oil

3 tablespoons hot water

Sea salt, to taste

1. Slice figs in half from stem to base, and set aside.

2. In a food processor, combine walnuts, pecans, Carob Extract™, and olive oil, and puree. As the processor is running, drizzle in hot water so that the mixture forms a thick paste similar in consistency to natural peanut butter. Season with sea salt, to taste.

3. Spoon about 1 teaspoon nut-butter mixture over each fig half and drizzle with extra Carob Extract™ if desired.

*Information about purchasing Carob Extract™ can be found in Appendix II: Products (page 235).

▶ SERVES 2

Drinks and Beverages

Anytime you start a new diet plan, it is nice to have a lot of taste and flavor options available to you, especially when you are just getting started. This will help to add diversity to your day in a simple and tasty way. Plus, there are plenty of us who have a routine of drinking coffee or black tea or soda, and these beverage suggestions can help to substitute for the old habits you are trying to kick. Included here are smoothies, which can spice up your snack or breakfast routine, or maybe even replace that milkshake that becomes tempting during the hot, summer months.

4 cups water

½ cup sliced peaches

1 cup mint leaves

4 chamomile tea bags

¼ cup peach nectar

1. Bring water to a gentle boil, and remove from heat. Add peaches, mint leaves, and tea bags, and steep for 4 to 5 minutes.

2. Remove tea bags, and let cool in refrigerator until chilled, about 1 hour.

3. Add peach nectar, stir, and serve over ice.

▶ SERVES 4

Sweet Basil and Ginger Tea

4 cups water

1 (2-inch) piece ginger, roughly chopped

¼ cup torn basil leaves

1 teaspoon agave nectar

1. Bring water to a boil with ginger, remove from heat, and add basil leaves. Let steep at least 3 minutes. Stir in agave and serve warm.

▶ SERVES 2

6 cups water

1 cup fresh mint

Juice and zest of 1 lime

2 teaspoons matcha powder

1 tablespoon honey

1. Heat water until it is almost at a boil. Add mint and lime juice and zest, and let steep, covered, for 5 minutes.

2. Spoon matcha powder into a heat-safe glass pitcher, and gradually pour water mixture over the matcha, whisking continuously. Strain the mint and zest out of the tea.

3. Add honey and serve.

▶ SERVES 4

featured ingredient

matcha

Matcha is a powdered form of green tea. Once tea leaves are sun-dried, they are finely ground and whisked into not-yet-boiling water. Matcha was originally used as a ceremonial tea in Japan, and has just recently become a popular trend in the United States. Because drinking matcha means ingesting all of the tea leaf instead of what is steeped from the leaves, you are consuming a greatly increased amount of antioxidants. Matcha can also be used in baked goods such as cookies and cakes.

Iced Chai Coffee

5 cups prepared coffee (**NS** substitute mix 3 tablespoons Carob Extract* into 5 cups 2 percent cow's milk)

1 whole clove

⅛ teaspoon ground nutmeg

¼ teaspoon dried ginger

⅛ teaspoon ground cardamom

2 tablespoons agave

½ cup 2 percent cow's milk, or more, to taste

1. Pour prepared coffee into a saucepan with the cloves, nutmeg, ginger, cardamom, and agave.

2. Warm ingredients over medium-low heat for 8 to 10 minutes, stirring occasionally. Remove and discard clove. Remove mixture from heat, and let cool. Place in the refrigerator until cold, about 1 hour.

3. Once chilled, pour into a large, glass pitcher, and add milk (add additional milk to suit your preference), and serve over ice in chilled glasses.

*Information about purchasing Carob Extract™ can be found in Appendix II: Products (page 235).

▶ SERVES 4

Tropical Kale Smoothie

1 cup frozen, diced pineapple

⅓ cup frozen, diced peach

½ frozen banana

¼ cup frozen kale

¾ cup 2 percent cow's milk

2 teaspoons agave

2 tablespoons Protein Blend™ Powder—Type B*

1. Place all ingredients in a blender, and blend until smooth, or use an immersion blender.

2. Serve chilled.

*Information about purchasing Protein Blend™ Powder—Type B can be found in Appendix II: Products (page 235).

▶ SERVES 4

 Type B

EAT RIGHT FOR YOUR TYPE PERSONALIZED COOKBOOK

1. Wash and dry vegetables. Cut off tough ends of the kale and carrots, and push kale, lemon, carrots, apples, and ginger through juicer one at a time.

2. Stir together and enjoy.

▶ SERVES 4

1 bunch kale
½ lemon
4 large carrots, peeled
4 apples
1 (3-inch) piece fresh ginger

tip: Vegetable juices will keep in the refrigerator for up to 3 days, but provide the best nutritional value when consumed immediately after juicing.

1. Combine all ingredients in a food processor and blend, or use an immersion blender. For easier blending, add liquid to the food processor first.

2. Serve chilled.

*Information about purchasing Protein Blend™ Powder—Type B can be found in Appendix II: Products (page 235).

▶ SERVES 2

1 frozen banana

1 teaspoon agave

2 tablespoons Protein Blend™ Powder—Type B*

1 cup 2 percent cow's milk

¼ cup frozen mango

1 tablespoon flaxseeds

1½ tablespoons almond butter

Berry Bonanza Smoothie (NS)

½ cup raspberries

½ cup pineapple

¾ cup blueberries

1 cup torn kale

1 cups 2 percent cow's milk

2 tablespoons almond butter

2 teaspoons agave

2 scoops Protein Blend™ Powder—Type B*

1. Combine all ingredients in a blender, and blend until smooth. Pour into 2 glasses and serve cold.

*Information about purchasing Protein Blend™ Powder—Type B can be found in Appendix II: Products (page 235).

▶ SERVES 2

Type B

EAT RIGHT FOR YOUR TYPE PERSONALIZED COOKBOOK

Desserts

What is a cookbook without desserts? The best way to stick to any kind of diet is to have realistic options for indulging your sweet tooth once in a while. Although these recipes sound indulgent, they are written to be as healthful as possible while still feeling like a satisfying dessert. Whenever possible use agave or molasses as sweeteners, include allowable grains, limit fats, and feel free to use chocolate.

1. Preheat oven to 350 degrees. Grease an 8" x 8" baking dish with nonstick spray and set aside.

2. In a large bowl, combine flours, arrowroot starch, cocoa powder, and sea salt. Set aside.

3. In a separate bowl, combine shaved chocolate and warm water, whisking until the chocolate fully melts (add 1 more tablespoon of water if necessary). Whisk in eggs, applesauce, butter, and agave. Add the chocolate mixture to the dry ingredients and stir to combine.

4. Pour into prepared pan, and bake for 30 minutes or until a cake tester or toothpick is inserted in the brownies and comes out clean.

5. Remove brownies from the oven, and turn off the heat. Pour chocolate chips over the top of the brownies, and place back into the oven for 2 to 3 minutes. Use an offset spatula to spread melted chips evenly across the top of the brownies. Let cool for 10 minutes.

6. Slice and serve. Brownies will stay in a cool, dry place overnight or in the freezer for up to 1 month.

▶ SERVES 8

tip: Light olive oil can be substituted here.

⅔ cup brown rice flour

⅓ cup millet flour

⅓ cup arrowroot starch

3 tablespoons cocoa powder

½ teaspoon sea salt

2 ounces melted 100 percent dark chocolate, shaved

3 tablespoons warm water

3 large eggs

¼ cup applesauce

4 tablespoons ghee, softened

½ cup agave

½ cup allergy-free chocolate chips

Nonstick cooking spray

featured ingredient

agave nectar

Agave is a natural sweetener derived from the agave plant, commonly found in the southwestern areas of America and in Mexico. Agave is most known for its role as the base ingredient of tequila. It can be used in baking and cooking in place of sugar; however the agave-to-sugar ratio is not 1:1 because it is a liquid. Agave has a mild taste akin to that of honey, but much less noticeable.

Cherry-Chocolate Fondue NS

fondue:

2 ounces 100 percent dark chocolate

2 tablespoons agave

1 cup cherry juice

1 tablespoon cherry jam

2 teaspoons ghee

1 cup diced pineapple

1 cup dried apricot

1 cup sliced apples

1. Shave chocolate into a mixing bowl.

2. In a saucepan, bring agave, juice, jam, and ghee to a simmer and remove from heat. Pour mixture over chocolate and stir to combine.

3. Serve with fruit for dipping.

▶ SERVES 6

Type B

1 cup whole almonds

½ cup quartered walnuts

½ cup halved macadamia nuts

2 teaspoons blackstrap molasses

1 teaspoon agave

½ cup chocolate chips

1 teaspoon large-grain sea salt

1. Preheat oven to 350 degrees.

2. Place almonds, walnuts, and macadamia nuts in a medium bowl, and toss to combine.

3. In a small saucepan, heat molasses and agave for 30 seconds over low heat, just until melted. Drizzle over nuts and toss. Very gently, spoon about 1 tablespoon nut clusters onto a wire cooling rack set over a baking sheet (if you do not have a wire cooling rack, you can spoon the same amount into mini cupcake pans coated with nonstick spray). Place wire rack or cupcake pan in the oven for 8 to 10 minutes.

4. Remove and let cool. Once cool, place in freezer for at least 10 minutes.

5. Melt chocolate in a double boiler. Note that water in the double boiler should never touch the base of the top pan to prevent burning.

6. Remove nut clusters from the freezer, and spoon melted chocolate over the top. Sprinkle evenly with sea salt, and freeze for an additional 10 minutes.

7. Serve cold or room temperature. Keep in an airtight glass container for up to 1 week or freeze for 1 month.

▶ SERVES 6

Creamy Berry Ricotta

16 ounces organic, part-skim ricotta cheese

⅛ teaspoon ground nutmeg

1 teaspoon lemon zest

2 teaspoons agave

¼ teaspoon sea salt

¾ cup sliced bananas

¾ cup sliced strawberries

1. In a medium-size bowl, stir together ricotta cheese, nutmeg, lemon zest, agave, and sea salt.

2. Use strawberries and banana to dip, or stir into ricotta mixture.

▶ SERVES 4

EAT RIGHT FOR YOUR TYPE PERSONALIZED COOKBOOK

Cocoa-Dusted Chocolate Truffles (NS)

8 ounces 100 percent dark chocolate

⅔ cup agave nectar

½ cup 2 percent cow's milk

⅛ teaspoon large-grain sea salt

¼ cup butter or ghee

3 tablespoons cocoa powder

1. Shave chocolate and place in a medium bowl. Warm agave nectar, milk, and salt in a saucepan set over low heat. Pour milk mixture over chocolate, whisking continuously until mixture becomes smooth.

2. Let the mixture come to room temperature, cover tightly, and refrigerate until chocolate is firm, about 2 to 3 hours.

3. Using a tablespoon or melon baller, scoop out truffles, and roll into balls (slightly smaller than golf ball size). Gently roll in cocoa powder and refrigerate until serving.

4. Store in an airtight container in the refrigerator for up to 1 week.

▶ SERVES 6

1. Preheat oven to 350 degrees. Grease a 9" x 11" baking dish, and set aside.

2. Combine flours, baking powder, and sea salt in a large bowl, and set aside.

3. Whisk whole eggs with ghee, and add to flour mixture, mixing until smooth and free of lumps.

4. In a clean, dry, glass bowl, beat egg whites until they form stiff peaks. Fold egg whites into batter, ⅓ at a time.

5. Pour batter into prepared baking dish, and bake for 12 to 15 minutes, until batter begins to firm.

6. While bars cook, combine all topping ingredients in a large bowl, mixing until well combined.

7. Remove bars from oven, and spoon topping mixture evenly over par-cooked bars. Return to the oven, and bake an additional 35 to 40 minutes or until a cake tester comes out clean.

8. Serve warm or room temperature. Bars will keep in a cool, dry place for 1 to 2 days, or in freezer for up to 1 month.

▶ SERVES 12

⅔ cup brown rice flour

¼ cup millet flour

¼ cup arrowroot flour

1 teaspoon baking powder

½ teaspoon sea salt

2 large eggs

4 tablespoons ghee, melted and cooled, plus more for greasing

2 large egg whites

topping:

½ cup fig jam

½ cup dried figs, cut into ½-inch dice

¼ cup agave

2 eggs, slightly beaten

1 egg white

2 teaspoons lemon zest

⅛ teaspoon ground nutmeg

⅛ teaspoon ground ginger

⅛ teaspoon ground cloves

2 tablespoons brown rice flour

1. Preheat oven to 350 degrees. Line an 11" x 17" baking sheet with parchment paper and set aside.

2. In a small bowl, pour hot water over cranberries to rehydrate them; let steep for 10 minutes.

3. In a large bowl, mix together flours, baking powder, salt, and almonds. Set aside.

4. In a separate bowl, whisk eggs, lemon zest, agave, and apricot jam. Add egg mixture to dry ingredients, stirring just until combined. Drain cranberries and pat dry. Toss cranberries into biscotti dough.

5. Gather dough into a ball and place on floured work surface. Gently roll dough with hands into a long, flat log, about the length of your baking sheet. Place on prepared baking sheet and bake for 30 minutes. Remove from oven and let cool 5 minutes. At this point, the cookie will have the texture of soft bread. Cut biscotti on the bias into ¾-inch slices, using a serrated knife. Place each slice flat on the baking sheet and bake for an additional 25 minutes, flipping once halfway through baking so that cookies are dry and crunchy all the way through.

6. Remove from oven and let cool on a wire rack. If using, heat chocolate morsels over a double boiler until melted and silky. Spoon chocolate over half of each cooled biscotti, and let the chocolate cool again.

7. Serve at room temperature. Store in a cool, dry place overnight or in freezer for up to 1 month.

▶ SERVES 12

¾ cup dried cranberries

1 cup amaranth flour

1½ cups brown rice flour, plus more for rolling

3 teaspoons baking powder

½ teaspoon fine-grain sea salt

1 cup slivered almonds

3 large eggs

1 teaspoon lemon zest

⅓ cup agave

⅓ cup apricot jam

½ cup chocolate morsels (optional)

Chocolate Chip Cookies NS

½ cup spelt flour

½ cup oat flour

1 teaspoon sea salt

½ teaspoon baking powder

½ teaspoon baking soda

½ cup ghee, softened

½ cup agave

1 tablespoon molasses

1 teaspoon vanilla

½ cup chocolate chips

1. Preheat oven to 350 degrees. Line a baking sheet with parchment paper and set aside.

2. In a large bowl, mix flours, baking powder, and baking soda.

3. In a separate bowl, beat softened ghee with agave, molasses, and vanilla until smooth and creamy.

4. Add ghee mixture to flour mixture and stir just until combined and free of lumps. Stir in chocolate chips, and spoon cookie dough by the tablespoon 2 inches apart on prepared baking sheet.

5. Bake 12 minutes in the center rack of the oven until cookies have golden-brown edges and are soft but firm to the touch.

6. Let cool on a wire rack or eat warm. Cookies stay in a cool dry place for 1 to 2 days or in the freezer up to 1 month.

▶ SERVES 12

EAT RIGHT FOR YOUR TYPE PERSONALIZED COOKBOOK

crust:

⅓ cup millet flour plus more for rolling

⅔ cup brown rice flour

½ teaspoon sea salt

3 tablespoons cold butter

4–5 tablespoons ice water

filling:

1 teaspoon lemon zest

¼ teaspoon sea salt

¼ teaspoon nutmeg

⅓ cup agave

¼ teaspoon ginger

2 cups (fresh or frozen) blueberries

topping:

¼ cup finely chopped walnuts

¼ cup brown rice flour

2 tablespoons butter or ghee

1 tablespoon agave

1. Preheat oven to 350 degrees.

2. In a large bowl, combine flours and sea salt. Cut cold butter into small pieces and add to flour mixture. Using a crossing motion with two butter knives or a pastry cutter, incorporate butter into the flour until the mixture resembles coarse cornmeal. Add water, 1 tablespoon at a time, until dough comes together but is not sticky. Gather dough in your hands and knead until it becomes smooth and pliable, using more flour if needed. Small pieces of butter should still be visible. Cover dough with plastic wrap and refrigerate 1 hour.

3. On a floured surface, roll out dough into a 12-inch circle. Carefully lift into a 9" pie dish, using a spatula to help you. Do not be discouraged if it falls apart; just push dough together. Set aside.

4. In a large bowl, stir together filling ingredients just until combined. Spoon into pie dish.

5. Make topping by combining walnuts and brown rice flour in a large bowl. Use your fingers to incorporate the butter into the dough. Stir in agave and sprinkle on top of blueberry filling.

6. Bake for 25 to 30 minutes.

▶ SERVES 4

Apple-Acai Charlotte

1 teaspoon ghee or butter plus more for greasing

1 teaspoon light olive oil

2 cups diced apples

¼ cup dried acai berries

¼ cup dry-toasted black walnuts

3 eggs

1 tablespoon 2 percent cow's milk

8 slices sprouted wheat bread, toasted

1. Preheat oven to 350 degrees. Grease sides and bottom of 2 (12-oz.) ramekins and set aside.

2. Heat ghee and olive oil in a medium skillet over medium heat. Add apples, acai berries, and walnuts, and cook 5 minutes. Set aside.

3. Whisk eggs and milk in a large, flat-bottomed bowl, and set aside.

4. Cut 6 toast slices to fit the bottom of prepared ramekins. Dip slices of bread in the egg wash as if making French toast. Line the bottom and edges of ramekins with the egg-soaked bread.

5. Divide apple mixture between ramekins, and top each 1 piece of toast soaked in egg wash.

6. Bake for 35 minutes or until golden brown.

7. Serve warm.

▶ SERVES 2

tip: If you cannot find dried acai berries, dried cranberries may be substituted in this recipe.

featured ingredient

acai

Acai, a tiny berry that is deep purple in color and only about an inch long, is cultivated from an acai palm tree in Central and South America. Like other berries, acai is rich in antioxidants and flavor.

EAT RIGHT FOR YOUR TYPE PERSONALIZED COOKBOOK

3 tablespoons ghee (melted and cooled) plus more for greasing

1 cup shredded carrot

¾ cup diced pineapple

1 cup brown rice flour

1 cup millet flour

¼ cup arrowroot starch

3 teaspoons baking powder

1 teaspoon salt

¼ teaspoon ground nutmeg

2 large egg yolks

1 cup finely chopped walnuts

½ cup agave

4 large egg whites

frosting:

½ cup 2 percent cow's milk

4 tablespoons agave

¼ teaspoon ground nutmeg

½ teaspoon ground ginger

⅛ teaspoon ground cloves

3 ounces 100 percent dark chocolate, grated

2 tablespoons ghee

2 tablespoons cocoa powder

¼ cup chopped walnuts, for garnish

1. Preheat oven to 350 degrees. Grease a 9-inch round cake pan and set aside.

2. Place shredded carrot and diced pineapple on separate paper towels to absorb excess liquid.

3. In a large bowl, combine dry ingredients, and set aside.

4. In a separate bowl, whisk together egg yolks, carrots, pineapple, walnuts, remaining 3 tablespoons ghee, and agave. Add to dry ingredients, stirring to combine.

5. In a dry, glass bowl, beat egg whites until stiff peaks form. Fold egg whites into batter, ⅓ at a time. Pour into prepared cake pan, and bake 35 to 40 minutes. Let cool on a rack in a cool, dry place for 30 minutes.

6. In the meantime, heat milk, agave, nutmeg, ginger, and cloves over low heat for 2 to 3 minutes. Place grated chocolate in a bowl with ghee. Pour milk mixture over chocolate, and whisk until smooth. Let cool completely. Add cocoa powder, and stir until mixture thickens.

7. Frost cake, and sprinkle with walnuts for garnish. Serve same day for best results, or store in a cool, dry place overnight or in the freezer for up to 1 month.

▶ SERVES 8

1. Preheat oven to 350 degrees. Grease 2 (9-inch-round) cake pans with 1 tablespoon ghee and set aside.

2. In a large bowl, combine matcha, flours, baking powder, salt, and cloves. Set aside.

3. In a separate bowl, whisk together lemon zest, agave, remaining 4 tablespoons ghee, eggs, egg yolk, and milk. Set aside.

4. Place egg whites in a dry glass, copper, or metal bowl and beat on high until egg whites form stiff peaks, and set aside.

5. Add wet mixture to dry mixture, and stir until well combined and lump-free. Using ⅓ of the egg white mixture at a time, fold whites gently into the batter.

6. Divide batter evenly between prepared cake pans. Bake in the middle rack of oven for 25 minutes, until cake is firm and cake tester comes out clean. Let cool in cake pans for 10 minutes, and remove to cool fully on wire cooling racks.

7. Prepare chocolate frosting by heating milk and agave in a small saucepan over low heat for 2 to 3 minutes. Place grated chocolate in a bowl with ghee. Pour hot milk over chocolate, and stir until smooth. Let cool completely. Add cocoa powder, and stir until mixture thickens.

8. Spread slightly less than half the frosting on the first layer of cake, and top with the second layer. Use an offset spatula to spread remaining frosting over the top of cake. Sprinkle with toasted macadamia nuts and chocolate morsels.

▶ SERVES 8

4 tablespoons ghee, melted and cooled, plus 1 tablespoon for greasing

1 tablespoon matcha powder

1½ cups brown rice flour

1 cup millet flour

3 teaspoons baking powder

½ teaspoon fine-grain sea salt

¼ teaspoon ground cloves

1 teaspoon lemon zest

½ cup agave

2 large eggs plus 1 yolk

⅓ cup 2 percent cow's milk

3 large egg whites

frosting:

½ cup 2 percent cow's milk

4 tablespoons agave

3 ounces 100 percent dark chocolate, grated

2 tablespoons ghee

2 tablespoons cocoa powder

⅔ cup chopped, toasted macadamia nuts

¼ cup allergy-free chocolate morsels

Upside-Down Almond Cake with Apricot Glaze (NS)

1 cup brown rice flour

½ cup millet flour

½ cup finely ground almond meal

2 teaspoons baking powder

½ teaspoon fine-grain sea salt

½ teaspoon lemon zest

4 large egg whites

2 large egg yolks

½ cup agave

4 tablespoons honey, divided

6 tablespoons ghee, softened

5 tablespoons 2 percent cow's milk

1 cup whole almonds

¼ cup sugar-free apricot jam

1. Preheat oven to 350 degrees. Grease a round 9-inch cake pan, line with parchment paper, and set aside.

2. In a large bowl, whisk together flours, almond meal, baking powder, and salt. Set aside.

3. In a dry, glass bowl, beat 4 egg whites with a hand mixer until stiff peaks are formed. Set aside.

4. Mix lemon zest, egg yolks, agave, 2 tablespoons honey, ghee, and milk in a small bowl, and add to dry mixture. Fold egg whites into batter, ⅓ at a time, just until combined.

5. Scatter almonds evenly on the bottom of prepared cake pan. In a small saucepan, warm remaining 2 tablespoons honey and apricot jam over low heat for 30 seconds. Glaze should be heated just enough to thin it out. Slowly pour glaze over almonds. Pour batter over almonds and bake for 40 minutes, or until a cake tester comes out clean.

▶ SERVES 8

EAT RIGHT FOR YOUR TYPE PERSONALIZED COOKBOOK

1. Combine all crêpe ingredients in a blender, and pulse until smooth and combined. Batter will be very thin. Let rest 1 hour in the refrigerator.

2. In the meantime, heat 1 teaspoon ghee in a skillet over medium heat. Sauté pear for 3 to 4 minutes or until slightly browned and tender. Add lemon zest, ginger, and apricot jam to hot skillet, and cook 30 seconds. Remove from heat and toss with fresh raspberries.

3. Preheat oven to 200 degrees.

4. Heat a large skillet over medium heat and melt 1 teaspoon ghee, brushing evenly to coat bottom of pan. Use a ¼-cup measure to scoop batter into pan. Quickly turn the pan in circular motions to spread the batter into a very thin layer. Let cook 1 minute or until the batter firms and edges lift slightly off the pan. Using an offset spatula, flip and cook 1 additional minute. Continue making crêpes until all batter is used. Stack finished crêpes in a slightly moist kitchen towel, and keep in the oven until ready to serve.

5. To serve, place a spoonful of chutney down the center of a crêpe, and roll up like a soft taco. Drizzle with chocolate syrup and serve warm.

*See Chocolate Syrup NS recipe (page 209).

▶ SERVES 4

tip: You can substitute cranberries for raspberries. Just cook with 1 tablespoon maple syrup.

Millet Crêpes with Raspberry Chutney and Chocolate Syrup NS

crêpes:

¾ cups millet flour

¼ cup spelt flour

½ teaspoon sea salt

1¼ cups 2 percent cow's milk

1 large egg

1 tablespoon plus 1 teaspoon ghee, melted and cooled

chutney:

1 teaspoon ghee

1 Bosc pear, diced

1 teaspoon lemon zest

½ teaspoon peeled and grated fresh ginger

¼ cup (no sugar added) apricot jam

1 teaspoon ghee

1 cup fresh raspberries, halved

Chocolate Syrup*

Banana-Based Ice Cream: 4 Ways

4 semi-ripened bananas, unpeeled

1. Freeze bananas overnight. Once frozen, peel and slice. Add to food processor and blend about 2 minutes, until bananas resemble creamy ice cream. Spoon into a bowl and serve. Add combinations below, for variety.

option 1: double chocolate

1 tablespoon cocoa powder
1 tablespoon agave
¼ cup mini dark chocolate chips

1. Add cocoa powder and agave to frozen bananas in the food processor and blend until smooth and creamy. Fold in chocolate chips and serve.

option 2: maple pecan/agave pecan

2 tablespoons maple syrup, divided (NS substitute agave)
⅓ cup chopped pecans
⅛ teaspoon sea salt

1. Toast pecans in a small skillet over medium heat. Add 1 tablespoon maple syrup and salt, and set aside to cool.

2. Add remaining maple syrup to food processor with frozen bananas and blend until smooth and creamy. Fold in cooled pecans and serve.

option 3: blueberry proberry

1 teaspoon Proberry 3™ liquid*
1 tablespoon agave
½ cup (fresh or frozen) blueberries

1. Add Proberry 3™ liquid and agave to bananas in food processor and blend until smooth and creamy. Stir in blueberries and serve.

▶ SERVES 4

tip: If bananas become too soft while adding other ingredients, simply store in a glass container and freeze for an additional 2 hours. Ice cream will keep in freezer for up to 1 week.

*Information on Proberry 3™ liquid can be found in Appendix II: Products (page 236).

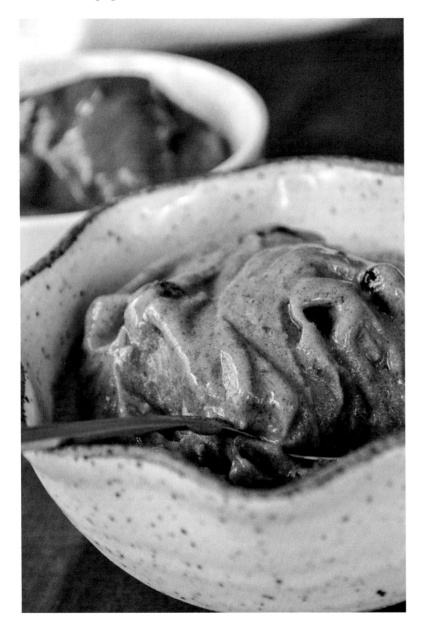

Ginger Rice Pudding (NS)

1 cup long-grain brown rice

½ teaspoon sea salt

3½ cups 2 percent cow's milk, divided

1 tablespoon fresh ginger, peeled and grated

⅛ teaspoon cardamom (optional)

⅛ teaspoon nutmeg

2 large egg yolks

2 tablespoons brown rice flour

1 tablespoon blackstrap molasses

1 tablespoon maple syrup

½ cup diced, dried pineapple (no sugar added)

1. In a medium saucepan, bring rice, ½ teaspoon sea salt, and 2 cups of milk to a boil. Reduce to a simmer, cover, and cook for 50 minutes.

2. In a small saucepan, heat remaining 1½ cups milk with ginger, cardamom, if using, and nutmeg over low heat until warm.

3. In a small bowl, whisk together egg yolks, flour, molasses, and maple syrup. Temper the egg mixture by very slowly adding a ladle of the warm milk to the eggs and whisking continuously.

4. Once the eggs have been warmed, add the mixture into the warmed milk and whisk over medium heat until the mixture is thick. The consistency should resemble yogurt when it is ready. Remove from heat and set aside.

5. When rice is cooked, add pineapple and milk mixture. Let cook an additional 3 to 5 minutes over low heat, stirring continuously. The rice pudding will be thick and creamy.

6. Serve warm.

▶ SERVES 4

EAT RIGHT FOR YOUR TYPE PERSONALIZED COOKBOOK

Stocks, Condiments, and Sauces

Herb Dressing

NS

¼ cup finely chopped fresh basil

2 tablespoons finely chopped fresh parsley

2 tablespoons finely chopped fresh chives

2 small cloves garlic, minced

½ cup extra virgin olive oil

⅔ cup fresh-squeezed lemon juice

½ teaspoon crushed red pepper flakes

Sea salt, to taste

1. Whisk herbs, garlic, olive oil, lemon juice, and red pepper in a small bowl, or pour ingredients in a resealable glass jar and shake vigorously to combine. Season with sea salt, to taste.

2. Store salad dressing in a glass jar or dispenser in the refrigerator for up to 1 week. Recipe can be doubled so you have it ready to go all week.

Citrus Dressing

NS

½ cup extra virgin olive oil

Juice of 2 lemons

Juice of 1 lime

2 tablespoons finely chopped cilantro

2 teaspoons agave

Sea salt, to taste

1. Whisk olive oil, lemon juice, lime juice, cilantro, and agave together in a small bowl, or pour ingredients in a resealable glass jar and shake vigorously to combine. Season with sea salt, to taste.

2. Store salad dressing in a glass jar or dispenser in the refrigerator for up to a week. Depending on how much dressing you might use, double this recipe so you have it ready to go all week.

Carrot-Ginger Dressing

2 medium carrots, peeled and chopped

1 tablespoon olive oil

1 (1-inch) piece fresh ginger, peeled

Sea salt, to taste

1. In food processor, pulse carrots, olive oil, and ginger until a smooth consistency is reached. If the mixture is too thick, add water, 1 tablespoon at a time.

2. Season with sea salt, to taste, and store in a glass container or dispenser in the refrigerator for up to 1 week.

Chocolate Syrup

1 cup agave

2 tablespoons cocoa powder

1. Whisk agave and cocoa powder vigorously in a bowl to incorporate. Store in a clean, glass dispenser or a glass container, to be drizzled over pancakes, fruit, or to add a special treat to smoothies.

2. Store in a cool, dry place for up to 2 weeks.

Turkey Stock (NS)

4 pounds turkey thighs and breast

3 large carrots, peeled and diced

1 celery root, peeled and diced

2 cloves garlic, peeled

1 Vidalia onion, chopped

4 quarts water

2 teaspoons sea salt

3 sprigs fresh thyme

3 sprigs fresh rosemary

5 sprigs parsley

2 bay leaves

1. Bring all ingredients to a gentle boil in a large stockpot. As the stock boils, use a large spoon to skim foam and impurities off the top and discard. Reduce to a simmer. After 3 hours, remove ingredients from stock and strain into a clean bowl or pot. Let cool (not more than 4 hours), then package and refrigerate. Store in glass containers in the refrigerator for up to 3 days or in the freezer for 2 months.

2. If you want to utilize the turkey meat for salad, casseroles, or to add to your soup, pick the meat off the bones after 1 hour of cooking, cool, and refrigerate for another use. Continue to cook the bones and vegetables. The stock will be lighter, but the meat will be viable for other uses (sandwiches, salads, in casseroles, pot pies, and so on).

Vegetable Stock

1. Heat olive oil in a large stockpot over medium heat. Sauté onion, celery root, parsnips, carrots, and fennel for 8 to 10 minutes, just until tender. Add water and remaining ingredients, and bring to a boil. Reduce heat to low, cover, and cook for 30 minutes. (Vegetable stock has a quick cooking time because vegetables give up their flavor quickly, as opposed to meats and bones.)

2. Strain stock into a clean pot, and store in the refrigerator for 3 to 5 days or in the freezer for 2 to 3 months.

2 teaspoons olive oil

2 onions, chopped

1 celery root, peeled and chopped

3 large parsnips, peeled and chopped

3 large carrots, peeled and chopped

2 fennel bulbs, chopped

4 quarts water

3 bay leaves

1 clove garlic, peeled

5 sprigs parsley

5 sprigs thyme

2 teaspoons sea salt

Basic Bread Crumbs (NS)

1. Toast slices of bread, let cool, and pulse in food processor to form coarse bread crumbs. To add flavor, add dried herbs such as parsley, rosemary, thyme, sage, and/or basil.

4 slices brown rice/millet or spelt bread

Beef Stock **NS**

3 bay leaves

4 sprigs fresh thyme

4 pounds beef bones

2 teaspoons olive oil

Sea salt, to taste

2 Vidalia onions, rough chopped

4 carrots, peeled and rough chopped

1 cup parsnips, peeled and rough chopped

4 quarts water, divided

2 cloves garlic, peeled

1 cup red wine

1. Preheat oven to 450 degrees.

2. Gather bay leaves and thyme in cheesecloth or use kitchen twine to secure them together. Set aside.

3. Place beef bones in a roasting pan and brush with olive oil and a dash of sea salt. Roast for 30 minutes.

4. Turn beef and add onions, carrots, and parsnips to the roasting pan. Bake for an additional 30 minutes. Remove and place beef bones and vegetables into a stockpot.

5. Deglaze roasting pan with 2 cups water, scraping up the bits off the bottom. If it is difficult to deglaze, simply place the baking dish over the burners on the stove over medium-low heat and continue scraping until all bits come up. Pour mixture into the stockpot. Add beef bones, remaining water, herbs, garlic, and red wine. Simmer 3 to 4 hours, skimming the top of the stock with a spoon while it cooks.

6. Strain stock into a clean pot and cool completely. Store in the refrigerator for 2 days or in the freezer for 2 months.

Useful Tools

Substitutions

An integral part of acclimating to your new diet is being able to fill the void created by your *Best Avoided* list. Below is a list of substitutions to help you along the way. A number of these are not direct substitutions but you will see from recipes in this book how they are adapted to work in place of the items on your *Best Avoided* list.

BREAD—As mentioned earlier, wheat is a *Neutral* grain for Type B but not desirable. The best option is to look for pure spelt, oat, or brown rice/millet breads. Many stores do not carry these breads, however they are accessible online. They are often less expensive to order online in bulk and store in the freezer. Bakers make flax, garlic-basil, and banana-walnut varieties, as well as bagels, rolls, hot dog buns, and even flatbreads, which are a perfect base for pizza. Just be sure to read labels carefully because many breads contain ingredients that may not work for your blood type.

PASTA—Spelt or brown rice pasta is fairly easy to come by these days, and found in most grocery stores. You want to look for a brand whose ingredients are nothing more than spelt or brown rice flour (or bran) and water. When cooking gluten-free (brown rice) pastas, the noodles will fall apart and become undesirably mushy if boiled too long. I recommend cooking rice pastas 3 to 4 minutes short of the recommended cooking time to ensure a good al dente texture for your pasta.

OIL—Vegetable, coconut, or soy oil is not recommended for most Type B diets, so what do you use in baking or cooking as an alternative? Olive oil is a *Beneficial* food for all Bs so you can stick with just that. Use light olive oil for baking so that there is not a pervasive olive taste in your baked goods. Of course, extra virgin olive oil is terrific for dressing salads or even a medium-heat stir-fry.

FLOUR—As a Type B, you have the best of both worlds: you can use the same flour combinations as both Type A and Type O, and both are used throughout this book. The approach to gluten-free baking used in this book is based on a combination of flours for texture and taste. Typically, you can use one of two combinations such as: brown rice flour, arrowroot starch, and millet. Brown rice flour can be swapped out for another hearty grain such as millet, amaranth, or quinoa. The other (not gluten-free) option is a spelt and oat flour mixture that works well as a base for most baked goods.

A great everyday baking mix for Type B is:
2 parts brown rice flour (⅔ cup for one batch)
1 part millet flour (⅓ cup for one batch)
1 part arrowroot starch flour (⅓ cup for one batch)
2 teaspoons baking powder
½ teaspoon sea salt

or:

2 parts spelt flour (⅔ cup for one batch)
1 part oat flour (⅓ cup for one batch)
2 teaspoons baking powder
½ teaspoon sea salt

Menu Planning

The following are suggestions to show you how to put the recipes in this book together to create weekly menus for you and your family. They are arranged in a way to keep a balanced diet, but feel free to mix and match as you see fit. If you plan to follow the menu exactly, read it thoroughly ahead of time so you can see where you would need to buy a little extra to account for leftovers, and where it's practical to plan/prep ahead. The purpose of menu planning is to make life as easy as possible by utilizing leftovers and planning more involved meals for weekends.

In addition to the list below, make sure you are drinking a minimum of six (8-oz.) glasses of water per day to stay properly hydrated.

MENU PLANNING TIPS:
- If you are working full-time or have difficulty preparing meals during the week, use time on the weekend to prepare snacks and

a few meals for the week by pre-washing vegetables and lettuce. This will significantly cut down on weekday duties. A few foods that stay well and that I always have are: Flax Crackers, Blackstrap Cherry Rice Granola, Spicy Rosemary-Nut Mix, and occasionally protein bars, like UniBar® Protein Bar.

- Leftovers are the most delightful time savers you could imagine. Pair them with a fresh salad, or toss in a soup, and they will become your best friend, too.
- When baking breads, muffins, or even sweet treats, freeze leftovers in sealable glass containers to keep them fresh. If you have Sweet Potato Muffins in the freezer, you can pop them in the oven or toaster oven at 200 degrees for 10 to 15 minutes, and they will be perfectly toasty and ready to eat. Frozen chocolate chip cookies are also delicious and don't require defrosting, just one of the great things about gluten-free flour.
- When making something like bruschetta, double the topping recipe, and reserve leftovers in a sealable glass container in the refrigerator for up to 1 week. That way you make it once, and it can be used as many times as you want it.

Four-Week Meal Planner
Week 1

Sunday

BREAKFAST: Pear-Rosemary Bread NS with sliced banana and raw walnuts

LUNCH: Ratatouille NS with sliced mozzarella cheese

SNACK: Cucumber slices with Curried Egg Salad NS

DINNER: Chili, Sans Tomatoes

Monday

BREAKFAST: Blackstrap-Cherry Rice Granola NS, rice cereal, and almond milk with green tea and fresh blueberries

LUNCH: Leftover Chili, Sans Tomatoes with mixed green salad dressed with lemon and olive oil

SNACK: Pear and Apple Chips and Spicy Rosemary-Nut Mix NS

DINNER: Lemon-Ginger Salmon NS with Brown Rice Salad NS

Tuesday

BREAKFAST: Scrambled Eggs with Blueberry-Macadamia Muffins and green tea

LUNCH: Raw Kale Salad with Zesty Lime Dressing **NS** and leftover Lemon-Ginger Salmon **NS**

SNACK: Flax Crackers **NS** and Summer Squash Salsa **NS**

DINNER: Crispy-Coated Turkey Tenders with Apricot Dipping Sauce and Sweet Potato Ragu **NS**

Wednesday

BREAKFAST: Homemade Turkey Breakfast Sausage **NS** with green tea and fresh raspberries

LUNCH: Raw Kale Salad with Zesty Lime Dressing **NS** and leftover Crispy-Coated Turkey Tenders with Apricot Dipping Sauce

SNACK: Pear and Apple Chips and Spicy Rosemary-Nut Mix **NS**

DINNER: Grilled Radicchio and Walnut-Spinach Pesto **NS**

Thursday

BREAKFAST: Blueberry-Macadamia Muffins with leftover Home-made Turkey Breakfast Sausage **NS** and green tea

LUNCH: Greens and Beans Salad **NS** with walnuts and crumbled feta

SNACK: Protein Blend™ Powder—Type B drink

DINNER: Tangy Pineapple and Beef Kabobs **NS** with Roasted Autumn Roots **NS**

Friday

BREAKFAST: Quinoa Muesli, banana slices, blueberries, and green tea

LUNCH: Leftover Greens and Beans Salad **NS** with leftover Tangy Pineapple and Beef Kabobs **NS**

SNACK: Carob–Walnut Butter–Stuffed Figs **NS**

DINNER: Mac and Cheese with Roasted Vegetables **NS** and Garlic–Creamed Spinach with Roasted Cauliflower **NS**

Saturday

BREAKFAST: Swiss Chard and Cremini Frittata **NS** with green tea and pineapple

LUNCH: ½ Bacon Grilled Cheese **NS** with Roasted Parsnip Soup **NS**

SNACK: Almond-Butter Rice Cakes with Mini Chips **NS**

DINNER: Seafood Paella **NS**

Week 2

Sunday

BREAKFAST: Cherry Scones NS with almond butter and green tea

LUNCH: Kidney Bean Stew

SNACK: Grilled Pineapple with Chocolate Syrup

DINNER: Moroccan Lamb Tagine

Monday

BREAKFAST: Breakfast Egg Salad NS with green tea

LUNCH: Mint and Red Pepper Tabbouleh NS with leftover Moroccan Lamb Tagine

SNACK: Homemade Applesauce

DINNER: Shredded Turkey Bake

Tuesday

BREAKFAST: Quinoa Muesli with sliced bananas and fresh blueberries

LUNCH: Leftover Shredded Turkey Bake with mixed greens dressed in olive oil and lemon

SNACK: Grilled Pineapple with Chocolate Syrup

DINNER: Beef and Shredded Cabbage Soup NS and Red Quinoa–Mushroom Casserole with Fried Egg NS

Wednesday

BREAKFAST: Swiss Chard and Cremini Frittata NS with sliced pineapple and green tea

LUNCH: Leftover Red Quinoa–Mushroom Casserole with Fried Egg NS

SNACK: Cheese Toast NS

DINNER: Parchment-Baked Snapper NS

Thursday

BREAKFAST: Broccoli-Feta Frittata NS with green tea

LUNCH: Navy Bean Hummus and Feta Sandwich NS

SNACK: Homemade Applesauce

DINNER: Rice and Bean Loaf NS with Spicy Collards NS and Baked Beans NS

Friday

BREAKFAST: Nut Butter–Granola Boats NS with green tea

LUNCH: Leftover Rice and Bean Loaf NS sandwiches

SNACK: Protein Blend™ Powder—Type B drink
DINNER: Spicy Seafood Stew **NS**

Saturday

BREAKFAST: Spelt Pancakes **NS** with scrambled eggs and green tea
LUNCH: Salmon-Filled Radicchio Cups **NS**
SNACK: Crispy Spring Vegetable Cakes **NS**
DINNER: Sweet Potato Gnocchi with Basil-Cranberry Sauce **NS** with grilled turkey cutlets

Week 3

Sunday

BREAKFAST: Pear-Rosemary Bread **NS** with a poached egg and green tea
LUNCH: Fish Fillet Sandwich **NS**
SNACK: Crudités and Creamy Goat Cheese Dip **NS**
DINNER: Turkey Mole Drumsticks with Whipped Sweet Potato Soufflé and Broccoli and Cabbage Slaw with Raisins **NS**

Monday

BREAKFAST: Creamy Banana–Nut Butter Smoothie **NS** and green tea
LUNCH: Leftover Turkey Mole Drumsticks and Broccoli and Cabbage Slaw with Raisins **NS**
SNACK: Unibar® Protein Bar
DINNER: Salmon and Bean Cakes with Cilantro-Cream Sauce **NS** and Spicy Roasted Mustard Greens with Feta **NS**

Tuesday

BREAKFAST: Pear-Rosemary Bread **NS** with scrambled eggs and green tea
LUNCH: Leftover Salmon and Bean Cakes with Cilantro-Cream Sauce **NS** and romaine lettuce dressed in lemon and olive oil
SNACK: Marinated Mozzarella Balls **NS** with Flax Crackers **NS**
DINNER: Hearty Slow-Cooker Turkey Stew **NS** with Sweet-and-Salty Brussels **NS**

Wednesday

BREAKFAST: Turkey Bacon–Spinach Squares **NS** and green tea
LUNCH: Leftover Hearty Slow-Cooker Turkey Stew **NS**

EAT RIGHT FOR YOUR TYPE PERSONALIZED COOKBOOK

SNACK: Unibar® Protein Bar

DINNER: Mushroom Soup with Parsley Pesto NS with Green Tea–Poached Turkey Tenderloins NS

Thursday

BREAKFAST: Blackstrap-Cherry Rice Granola NS and yogurt with green tea and fresh blueberries

LUNCH: Shredded leftover Green Tea–Poached Turkey Tenderloins NS with cranberries and walnuts over spinach greens with olive oil and lemon

SNACK: Marinated Mozzarella Balls NS with Flax Crackers NS

DINNER: Fig-Stuffed Turkey Breasts with Roasted Sweet Potatoes with Fried Sage NS

Friday

BREAKFAST: Homemade Turkey Breakfast Sausage NS with green tea and fresh raspberries

LUNCH: Leftover Fig-Stuffed Turkey Breasts with Roasted Sweet Potatoes with Fried Sage NS over Raw Kale Salad with Zesty Lime Dressing NS

SNACK: Unibar® Protein Bar

DINNER: Spiced Lamb with Wild Mushrooms NS with Broccoli–Northern Bean Soup NS

Saturday

BREAKFAST: Spinach-Pepper Soufflé NS and green tea

LUNCH: Crunchy Vegetable Spring Rolls with Sweet Cherry Dip NS

SNACK: Farmer Cheese and Beet-Endive Cups NS

DINNER: Spring Pesto Pasta NS with grilled halibut

Week 4

Sunday

BREAKFAST: Savory Herb and Cheese Bread Pudding NS

LUNCH: Navy Bean Hummus and Feta Sandwich NS

SNACK: Tropical Fruit Salad with Mint and Lime Dressing NS

DINNER: Sweet Potato Shepherd's Pie NS with Roasted Escarole NS

Monday

BREAKFAST: Maple-Sausage Scramble NS and green tea

LUNCH: Leftover Sweet Potato Shepherd's Pie **NS**

SNACK: Roasted Cauliflower Bruschetta **NS**

DINNER: Baked Mahimahi with Crunchy Fennel Salad **NS** and Herbed Quinoa **NS**

Tuesday

BREAKFAST: Sweet Potato Muffins with Carob Drizzle with almond butter and green tea

LUNCH: Baked Falafel **NS** and Roasted-Eggplant Greek Salad **NS**

SNACK: Tropical Fruit Salad with Mint and Lime Dressing **NS**

DINNER: Greek Lamb Burgers **NS** and Broccolini with Crispy Walnut Bacon **NS**

Wednesday

BREAKFAST: Nut Butter–Granola Boats **NS** with yogurt and green tea

LUNCH: Leftover Broccolini with Crispy Walnut Bacon **NS** wrapped in Boston Bibb lettuce with goat cheese

SNACK: Crudités and Navy Bean Hummus **NS**

DINNER: Turkey-Ginger Stir-Fry **NS** with Carrot-Ginger Soup **NS**

Thursday

BREAKFAST: Breakfast Egg Salad **NS** with green tea

LUNCH: Leftover Carrot-Ginger Soup **NS** and ½ Bacon Grilled Cheese **NS**

SNACK: Roasted Cauliflower Bruschetta **NS**

DINNER: Pasta Carbonara with Asparagus **NS** with Greens and Beans Salad **NS**

Friday

BREAKFAST: Sweet Potato Muffins with Carob Drizzle with almond butter and green tea

LUNCH: Leftover Greens and Beans Salad **NS** with walnuts and fresh mozzarella

SNACK: Crudités and Creamy Goat Cheese Dip **NS**

DINNER: Fish Tacos with Bean and Crunchy Fennel Slaw **NS**

Saturday

BREAKFAST: Oat Crêpes and green tea

LUNCH: Melted Mozzarella–Onion Soup **NS**

SNACK: Baked Grapefruit

DINNER: Turkey Pot Pie with Crunchy Topping **NS**

Tools

YOU CAN FIND the following helpful tools on our website page at http://www.4yourtype.com/cookbooks.asp. Download these PDFs and print them from your computer.

- Food Journal
    Keep track of every meal with this handy log.

- Tracking Your Progress
    This is an additional log to help you focus on your goals.

- Shopping List
    Make your shopping trip easy with this list of *Beneficial* foods for your type.

TYPE B SHOPPING LIST
Produce:

Beets	Ginger	Cranberries
Broccoli	Kale	Grapes
Cabbage	Peppers	Pineapple
Carrots	Sweet potatoes	Watermelon
Eggplant	Bananas	

Baking:

Brown rice flour	Spelt flour	Agave
Millet flour	Baking powder	Molasses
Oat flour	Sea salt	

Dairy:

Butter	Eggs	Mozzarella
Cottage cheese	Feta cheese	Ricotta
Cow's milk	Goat cheese	Yogurt

Meat/Seafood:

Cod	Lamb	Turkey
Flounder	Mahimahi	Venison
Halibut	Salmon	

Miscellaneous:

Olive oil	Navy beans	Ginger tea
Almonds	Oat bread	Green tea
Almond butter	Spelt bread	Peppermint tea
Walnuts	Cayenne pepper	
Kidney beans	Parsley	

Please note: This shopping list only highlights the most frequently used *Beneficial* and some *Neutral* foods for Type B. For a complete list of *Beneficials*, *Neutrals*, and *Avoids*, refer to *Eat Right 4 Your Type*, the *Blood Type B Food, Beverage, and Supplement Lists*, or your SWAMI personal nutrition plan.

Time to Think Green

MICHEL NISCHAN IS a sustainable chef, cookbook author, and connoisseur of local, healthy food. He wrote in one of his books, *Sustainably Delicious: Making the World a Better Place, One Recipe at a Time*, "Where there is flavor, there are nutrients, and where there are nutrients, there is health." It is well known by chefs around the globe that the best food comes from the freshest ingredients, and nothing is fresher than a tomato grown in your own backyard or at the local farm. When you meander through your local farmers market and browse fruits and vegetables picked at their peak of freshness, the smells, touch, and tastes become infinitely more vibrant than a similar stroll through the supermarket. If you start any meal with fresh, local, whole-food ingredients, almost anything you make will be the best-tasting food and the best for your health.

Below you can find a few highlights on buying organic, avoiding toxins in your kitchen, and shopping for the freshest fruits and vegetables.

Quick Review of the Terms

Whenever possible, buy organic food and grass-fed beef. Why? Conventional fruits and vegetables are sprayed with harmful chemicals such as herbicides, pesticides, and insecticides. The chemicals used in these substances can disrupt hormones, and potentially cause cancer, allergies, asthma, and other health issues. Meat, dairy, and poultry raised conventionally exist in poor conditions and are fed for the purpose of fast weight gain, which is taxing to their health. As a result, animals are given antibiotics, which end up in the meat you buy at the grocery store. In addition, some animals are put on hormones to bulk up their bodies, making their meat artificially larger and, therefore, more desirable to consumers' eyes.

To review, here are a few definitions to sort out some of the confusion.

100 Percent USDA Certified Organic—This means that the product you purchase must contain ONLY organic ingredients, minus water and salt. Knowing the abbreviation USDA is an easy way to identify foods that are 100 percent certified organic.

Organic—Products must contain a minimum of 95 percent organic ingredients. Each ingredient within the product that is organic must also be labeled as such.

Made with Organic Ingredients—This label indicates that 70 percent or more ingredients contained in the product are organic. These products also cannot predominantly display the word *organic*.

Natural—The product has to contain no artificial ingredients or added color, and is processed in a way that does not fundamentally alter the product.

No Hormones—This term can only be used for beef. Poultry and pork are not allowed to be raised using hormones, so the label is unnecessary.

Grass-Fed—This term applies to animals that are solely fed grass and hay.

Free-Range—This indicates that animals are allowed access to the outside. This label is tricky, however, because there are a large number of farms that are keeping their animals in poor conditions but allowing a tiny space for "outdoor access" in order to be labeled "free-range." How do you determine if eggs are coming from humane farms? Check out http://www.cornucopia.org/organic-egg -scorecard for a scored list of farms.

Tips for Buying Local and Organic
Choosing Food That Is in Season

This phrase is tossed around a lot, but what is the benefit of eating "in season"? Taste. Obviously, it also has a significant environmental impact, but the difference between eating a fresh apple off a tree versus a genetically modified apple from the grocery store is striking enough to convince even the harshest skeptics. Eating in season also ensures that you are rotating the kinds of fruits and vegetables in your diet, and as a result, the nutrients.

There is nothing more refreshing than fresh watermelon in the summer or roasted sweet potatoes in the fall. Make a habit of eating only the best by choosing local, organic food that is in season.

Where to Find Fresh Food in Season?

Look for local listings indicating farm stands or farmers markets. Most farms are also happy to show you around if you want to stop by for a visit or take your children to see how food is grown and raised. A terrific resource for finding local food is: www.localharvest.org. Just fill out your city/state and you will be provided with a listing of local and organic food happenings. I always feel that eating in season is more satisfying to my body and palate.

Local or Organic?

Sometimes we have to make the choice between eating local or organic food, and it can be confusing. Local food is terrific because of its freshness and limited impact on the environment; it does not have to be shipped all the way from Chile to get to your table. Food that is organic, however, is grown without harmful chemicals that are detrimental to your health but also negatively impact our environment. In an ideal world we wouldn't have to choose between organic and pesticide-free, but sometimes that is the choice that we are faced with as consumers. Thankfully, many independent local farms practice organic farming, which can limit the need for these choices.

Healthy Choices on a Budget?

At some point, we all have to watch what we spend on everything, including food. The number-one tip I have for maintaining a healthy diet on a budget is prioritizing. If you are eating right for your blood type, you will be cutting out extras like potato chips, soda, prepared dips, cookies, and most overly processed foods. This alone will start to make room in your budget for healthier alternatives. Additionally, buying food in season is far less expensive than buying those same foods out of season. A pint of organic blueberries in the middle of the winter can cost up to $6.99; the same pint at the farmers market in the summer can go as low as $2.99. When stocking up on grains or nuts, be savvy and buy in bulk. Nuts contain fats that, if left in your pantry, could spoil quickly. To keep them fresh, store excess nuts in the freezer. Buying in bulk also means you are cutting down on the cost and waste of excess packaging, which you definitely pay for.

Finally, prioritizing your organic purchases will save you a bundle. There are twelve fruits and vegetables that carry the most pesticide residue; therefore, buying these ingredients organic should take priority. (See the foods on the Dirty Dozen listed below.) If you are on a budget, don't cut out these foods entirely, simply cut back how many you buy in one trip. Try to pick one or two ingredients that you must buy organic and supplement them with produce known to carry the lowest levels of pesticides, also known as the Clean Fifteen.

Dirty Dozen/Clean Fifteen

Below is a list of the Dirty Dozen*. Try to buy these organic as often as possible to reduce your pesticide exposure.

1. Apples
2. Celery
3. Strawberries
4. Peaches
5. Spinach
6. Nectarines—imported
7. Grapes—imported
8. Sweet bell peppers
9. Potatoes
10. Blueberries—domestic
11. Lettuce
12. Kale/Collard greens

Listed here are the Clean Fifteen*, a list of produce that has the smallest traces of pesticides and are therefore safest to buy in their conventional form. If it is possible, however, choosing organic is always better for yourself and the environment.

1. Onions
2. Sweet corn (*Avoid* for B)
3. Pineapples
4. Avocado (*Avoid* for B)
5. Asparagus
6. Sweet peas
7. Mangoes

8. Eggplant
9. Cantaloupe—domestic
10. Kiwi
11. Cabbage
12. Watermelon
13. Sweet potatoes
14. Grapefruit
15. Mushrooms

*Dirty Dozen and Clean Fifteen taken from the Environmental Working Group website, www.ewg.org.

Safe Food Storage

The first question is, what is safe? As most of us are aware, there is a chemical in most plastics called BPA (Biphenol-A), which when ingested acts as a hormone disrupter. Studies recently conducted report that BPA negatively affects hormone levels, which can lead to obesity as well as problems with thyroid function and the risk of certain cancers.

Where Is BPA Found?

BPA is a compound found in consumer products such as plastic containers, water bottles, plastic wrap, cans, and some cartons. Plastics labeled 3, 6, or 7 for recycling purposes often contain BPA.

What Makes BPAs Leach into Our Food?

Cans contain BPA in their lining. Therefore, when a can contains foods with high levels of acidity (like tomatoes), there is a greater likelihood that BPA will seep into the food it contains. Foods with high acidity also affect plastics, but a drastic change in the temperature of plastics (like freezing or being left in a warm car) will have the same leaching effect.

How Do I Avoid Them?

Thankfully, it is getting easier and easier to avoid BPAs, mostly because they are being banned by the government in most products for children. Additionally, the more we know about the harmful effects of BPA, the more demand there is in the market for products that are free of this harmful chemical. There are many companies putting BPA-free products on the market. A terrific alternative to canned tomatoes are products packaged by Tetra Pak; all of their packaging is BPA-free. Additionally, look for foods packaged in glass jars as opposed to cans or plastics.

What Should Be Done About Buying Food in Plastic/Cans?

The best way to purchase food is fresh, in glass, or in Tetra Pak cartons. Meats and seafood that are packaged by your butcher in plastic can be swapped out at home for further storage. If you feel inclined, however, let your butcher know you would prefer your food wrapped in paper. If enough people speak up, a change will certainly happen.

How Do I Pack Safe School Lunches?

Traditionally, kids' lunch boxes and plastic bottles contained BPAs. The good news is that there are an increasing number of BPA-free options available; you just have to look for them. Due to recent studies about the adverse affects of BPA on health, most companies are trying to or are required by law to switch to BPA-free packaging. That being said, glass containers with sealable lids are available in many different sizes and are another great alternative to plastic.

NOTE: Get kids involved, so they start learning young. Let them help you in the process of preparing and packing their lunches. This allows them to learn about healthier nutrition. Choose fun, nontoxic snack packs for them to store their lunches.

Cleaning up the Kitchen

What's Wrong with Chemicals?

Traditional household cleaners contain chemicals such as alkylphenols, alkylphenol ethoxylates, ammonia, chlorine, and diethanolamine, just to name a few. These chemicals can cause allergies, skin irritation, asthma, and potentially much more serious health problems. Avoiding these chemicals and others in our environment is pretty much impossible, but what we can do is become aware of where they exist and limit our exposure as much as possible. The first step is cleaning out your detergents, bleach, disinfectant sprays, or wipes along with any other cleaning products.

Is It More Expensive to Use Natural Cleaners?

If you're smart about it, it doesn't have to be. In fact, cleaning with natural products can actually be less expensive. For example, vinegar is mentioned below as a replacement to some cleaning products. A generic brand of vinegar is about $0.02/ounce, and a little definitely goes a long way.

What Are Some Household Products That Can Clean Well?

The best non-toxic cleaners are vinegar, baking soda, lemon juice, and club soda. Vinegar is a natural disinfectant and, believe it or not, deodorizer. You can use it to clean your floors, countertops, sinks, and any surface that needs cleaning. Baking soda mixed with water is slightly abrasive and can be used to clean stainless steel and carpets, and acts as a fabric softener and deodorizer.

Additional Information on the Blood Type Diet

Discover Your Blood Type

It is difficult to begin a diet based on blood type if you are not aware of your own type. In Europe, blood type is something almost everyone knows, but here in the United States, unless we need a transfusion, we can go our entire lives without knowing what blood type we are. Here are several simple ways to find out your type:

Donate blood. Not only are you providing a critical service to the community, but this is a free and simple way to find out what blood type you are. To find your local donation center, visit the American Red Cross website's Give Blood page (www.redcrossblood.org).

Purchase a blood typing test kit at D'Adamo Personalized Nutrition (www.4yourtype.com), under Books and Tests. The kit is inexpensive and simple to do in your own home.

Next time you visit your doctor for a blood workup, ask him or her to add blood type to the blood-draw protocol.

Secretor Status

In this book we also address Secretor Status, tagging each recipe to indicate if it is appropriate for both Secretors and Non-Secretors. If you do not know your Secretor Status, you can purchase a Secretor Status Test Kit from D'Adamo Personalized Nutrition (www.4yourtype.com).

Center of Excellence in Generative Medicine

The Center of Excellence (COE) in Generative Medicine is a collaboration between Dr. Peter D'Adamo and the University of Bridgeport to create a frontiers-focused biomedical initiative without parallel in any other medical school. The COE combines patient care, clinical research, and hands-on teaching opportunities for students in UB's Health Sciences program. It is also home to Dr. Peter D'Adamo's clinical practice. For information and appointments for either private practice patients or Clinic Shift patients, please contact:

Center of Excellence in Generative Medicine
115 Broad Street
Bridgeport, CT 06604
(203) 366-0526
www.generativemedicine.org/

D'Adamo Personalized Nutrition®—North American Pharmacal, Inc.

For information on the Blood Type Diets, individualized supplements, and testing kits, please contact:

North American Pharmacal, Inc.
213 Danbury Road
Wilton, CT 06897
International: (203) 761-0042
Toll-Free USA: (877) 226-8973
Fax: (203) 761-0043
www.4yourtype.com

www.dadamo.com—For All Things Peter D'Adamo

One of the longest running websites on the Internet, www.dadamo.com is the home page for the community of netizens who follow the work of Dr. Peter D'Adamo. This easy-to-navigate site is chockful of helpful tools, blogs, and one of the warmest, most welcoming chat forums to be found. Newbies are welcome to this moderated, family-friendly community.

Products

Here is information about products designed by Dr. D'Adamo that were mentioned in this book and where you can find them:

Protein Blend™ Powder—Type B

We created a specific protein powder to benefit the individual needs of each blood type. Type B has a high protein content based on rice protein and egg whites, and contains no sugar.

Protein Blend™ Powder can be purchased online at: www.4yourtype .com. Simply click "Specialty Products" and scroll down to find Bars and Shakes.

Unibar® Protein Bar

The Unibar® is the healthy snack you don't have to feel guilty about! Designed for all blood types, including Secretor and Non-Secretor, the Unibar® is ideal as a meal replacement, clean-fuel workout bar, or nutritious snack for a burst of energy between meals.

Chocolate Cherry (15 grams of protein) and Blueberry Almond (13 grams of protein) Unibar®s can be purchased online at: www.4yourtype .com. Simply click "Specialty Products" and scroll down to Bars and Shakes.

Carob Extract™

This delicious, irresistible syrup made from the carob bean is *Beneficial* for all blood types for easing digestive discomfort as well as coping with fatigue. It's so good that 1 teaspoon a day won't be enough. Use as a topping on crêpes, ice cream, muffins, and even cereals.

Carob Extract™ can be purchased online at: www.4yourtype.com. Simply click "Specialty Products" and scroll down to Bars and Shakes.

Proberry 3™ Liquid

Developed for immune support, Proberry 3™ comes in both capsules and liquid . . . but after tasting the liquid you will be hooked. I drink it by the teaspoonful when I have a cold, or I drizzle it in smoothies, mix in ice cream, or stir into tea for a tasty boost of antioxidants.

Proberry 3™ can be purchased online at: www.4yourtype.com. Simply click "Right for All Types," then "Immune Support" and scroll down to find Proberry 3™ liquid.

For a complete list of all products formulated by Dr. Peter J. D'Adamo, go to www.4yourtype.com.

SWAMI© Personalized Nutrition Software Program

Dr. D'Adamo developed the SWAMI software to harness the power of computers and artificial intelligence, using their tremendous precision and speed to help tailor unique one-of-a kind diets.

From its extensive knowledge base, SWAMI can evaluate over 700 foods for over 200 individual attributes (such as cholesterol level, gluten content, presence of antioxidants, etc.) to determine if that food is either a superfood or toxin for you. It provides a personalized kind diet in an easy to read, friendly format. For more information about SWAMI, you can go to www.4yourtype.com.

References

1. Bob's Red Mill. Bob's Red Mill Natural Foods. www.bobsredmill.com. Accessed May 2013.

2. D'Adamo, Peter J., and Whitney, Catherine. *Eat Right 4 Your Blood Type*. New York: G. P. Putnam's Sons, 1996.

3. D'Adamo, Peter J., and Whitney, Catherine. *Live Right 4 Your Blood Type*. New York: G. P. Putnam's Sons, 2001.

4. "EWG's Shopper's Guide to Pesticides in Produce." Environmental Working Group, www.ewg.org, 2011.

5. "Food Labeling/Organic Foods." Usda.gov. United States Department of Agriculture, www.usda.gov, May 10, 2011.

6. Healthy Child, Healthy World. October 23, 2011. www.healthychild.org.

7. Mateljan, George. "The World's Healthiest Foods." www.whfoods.com. Accessed May 2013.

8. Nischan, Michel, and Goodbody, Mary. *Sustainably Delicious: Making the World a Better Place, One Recipe at a Time*. New York: Rodale Books, 2010.

Acknowledgments

PETER J. D'ADAMO

It is with great pleasure to share with the readers of *Eat Right 4 Your Type* and followers of my work on the Blood Type Diet and my continuing explorations in the area of personalized medicine the *Eat Right 4 Your Type Personalized Cookbook* series. There are many people I would like to thank, as this was a group effort.

My deep appreciation to Berkley Books, a division of Penguin Group (USA), as my longtime publisher; in particular, my editor, Denise Silvestro, whose personal belief in these cookbooks brought them from their original e-book format to where we are today; publisher, Leslie Gelbman; Allison Janice, who coordinated the production efforts; Pam Barricklow, the managing editor; and the entire Berkley team who worked on these books. I would also like to thank my dedicated agent, Janis Vallely, whose encouragement, guidance, and tenacity have made this book possible.

A very special thanks to Kristin O'Connor, whose culinary skills, combined with her depth of knowledge of and belief in the Blood Type Diet, have allowed us to develop delicious, nutritious recipes that are right for your type.

A special nod of appreciation for our team at North American Pharmacal and Drum Hill, who worked on these books as they were being developed, especially Bob Messineo, Wendy Simmons-Taylor, Ann Quasarano, John Alvord, Emily D'Adamo, and Angela Bergamini.

As always, I am grateful to my wife and partner, Martha Mosko D'Adamo, for her unwavering support and for the role she played in shepherding these books into existence; and to my two daughters, Claudia and Emily, who share a deep passion for this work and for a well-cooked meal.

A final thanks to the hundreds of thousands of readers and followers who have shared this journey with me. I am encouraged and fortified by your continuing dedication to your personal health and well-being, and I am humbled by your trust and commitment to this work.

KRISTIN O'CONNOR

I am so fortunate to have such a huge arena of support; I truly could not have done it without any of you.

First, of course is Dr. Peter D'Adamo, the science behind this effective diet. I will always respect your brilliant mind and interest in making this world a healthier place. To my mother, Susan O'Connor, for being the reason I had so much faith in this diet, teaching me how to cook, supporting my every move, and being there by my side while testing all six hundred recipes! To my father, Kevin O'Connor, who sees more potential in me than anyone I've ever met, guided me in the basics of photography, and taught me to have the courage to put myself out there over and over again. My brother, Dr. Ryan O'Connor, for valuing my accomplishments and always sharing in the joy of my success as if it were his own . . . and being a very willing recipe-testing guinea pig! To my grandparents Mike and Ellie DeMaio, thank you for being my cheerleaders, and for providing encouragement and unconditional support.

A huge thank you to David Domedion for utilizing his expertise to meticulously edit every recipe. Thank you to Chris Bierlein for his incredible talent, kind spirit, and generosity with shooting and editing our gorgeous cover photos. We were privileged to work with both of you.

Heather Rahilly, whose friendship kept me sane and whose intellect kept me in the race, thank you for being the most thorough attorney I could ask for! To my friends, who are all like family to me, for selflessly offering help in any way they could: Annie Gaffron, Mandy Geisler, Latha Chirunomula (along with Padma and Pushpavathi for teaching me the basics of South Indian cooking), Jennifer Eastes, Iwona Lacka, and the Metwallys.

Thank you to Tim Macklin for being my very patient mentor, and a great source of knowledge and encouragement. Thanks to Danielle Boccher, Scott Olnhausen, and the rest of my pals at Concentric! Special thanks to Dr. Peter Bongiorno and Dr. Pina LoGiudice for taking me under their wing when I was just a little fledgling cook wanting to make a difference.

Thank you to Kate Fitzpatrick and Ann Quasarano, whose dependability and efforts at getting our book out there in the public eye was very much appreciated. To Stephen Czick for his hours of editing and support, and Wendy Simmons-Taylor for all her patience with styling these books.

Thanks to Martha D'Adamo and the team at Drum Hill Publishing for giving me the opportunity to work on these cookbooks, which I very much love and believe in.

And finally, a very special thank you to Craig Anderson for taking a chance on me at the very beginning and opening the doors to my dreams.

PETER J. D'ADAMO

A second-generation naturopathic doctor, Dr. D'Adamo has been practicing naturopathic medicine for more than thirty years. Best known for his research on human blood groups and nutrition, Dr. D'Adamo is also a well-respected researcher in the field of natural products and a Distinguished Professor of Clinical Sciences at the University of Bridgeport. He is the founder and director of the Center of Excellence in Generative Medicine, a clinical, academic and research institute, which also houses his private clinical practice located in a beautifully restored Victorian house on the campus of the University of Bridgeport overlooking the Long Island Sound. Dr. D'Adamo is the recipient of the 1990 AANP Physician of the Year Award for his role in the creation of the *Journal of Naturopathic Medicine*. Dr. D'Adamo's series of books are *New York Times* Bestsellers and Book-of-the-Month-Club selections. He was named the "Most Intriguing Health Author of 1999," and his first book, *Eat Right 4 Your Type*, was voted one of the "Ten Most Influential Health Books of All Time" by media industry analysts. Publishers Weekly called his third book, *Live Right 4 Your Type*, "A comprehensive and fascinating theory that has been meticulously researched." His books have been translated in to sixty-five languages, and there are over 7 million copies of his books worldwide.

KRISTIN O'CONNOR

Kristin O'Connor has made it her life's work to create food that is irresistibly tasty and healthy, a combination she hopes will inspire people to love good healthy food and encourage them to make it a lifelong habit. In doing so, she created NourishThis.com—a website with recipes, articles, and tips on eating well and living green; volunteers for Healthy Child, Healthy World—a nonprofit that educates parents about nutritional and environmental issues affecting their children; and presented at The Kids Food Festival in Bryant Park, New York City. She has worked for a Food Network and Cooking Channel production company as an associate producer on many of their shows, was an above-the-line catering chef for a lead actor on a major motion picture, and is now working as a private celebrity chef. Kristin continues to volunteer for nonprofit organizations that promote a healthy diet and environment and hopes to continue her career as a cookbook author in the future.